THE PATIENT AS THE CENTER

Integrating Psychodynamic Approaches with Other Mental Health Treatments

WILLIAM G. HERRON
Bergen New Bridge Medical Center

RAFAEL ART. JAVIER
St. John's University
New York University Postdoctoral Program in
Psychotherapy and Psychoanalysis
Object Relations Institute for
Psychotherapy and Psychoanalysis

ROWMAN & LITTLEFIELD
Lanham • Boulder • New York • London

Executive Acquisitions Editor: Mark Kerr
Assistant Acquisitions Editor: Sarah Rinehart
Sales and Marketing Inquiries: textbooks@rowman.com

Published by Rowman & Littlefield
An imprint of The Rowman & Littlefield Publishing Group, Inc.
4501 Forbes Boulevard, Suite 200, Lanham, Maryland 20706
www.rowman.com

86-90 Paul Street, London EC2A 4NE

British Library Cataloguing in Publication Information Available

Library of Congress Cataloging-in-Publication Data Available

ISBN 978-1-5381-6326-9 (cloth)
ISBN 978-1-5381-6327-6 (paperback)
ISBN 978-1-5381-6328-3 (ebook)

For all my daughters: Judith, Rachel, Lia, Mara, Abigail, Allison
—William G. Herron

*To the memory of my colleague and good friend, Herb Gingold, who
personified in his actions the true meaning and importance of inclusivity in
what and how we do what we do. It is also dedicated to CERCCL at the
New York University Postdoctoral Program for their excellent work and
determination in addressing this very issue in psychoanalytic training.*
—Rafael Art. Javier

Brief Contents

Contents

Acknowledgments

This book is a reaction to my many years of being a practicing psychotherapist. I have learned a lot, felt a lot, and am grateful to be still practicing. I believe therapists must go with the flow of patient needs and support services that do that effectively. Currently that means having a strong voice and doing what works, which translates into integrative psychotherapy. This book was made possible by the strong voice of Rafael Javier, my frequent collaborator; the tuned-in editors at Rowman and Littlefield; my daughter Lia, who enables me to appear computer literate; and the many patients who trusted me with a significant role in their lives.

—William G. Herron

Just a word of thanks to my patients for allowing me to witness their courageous involvement in their therapeutic journey. In their attempts to find meaning in their life journey, they forced a conversation and exploration of their multiple identities of their lived experience that required me to remain impartially open and receptive to witness and participate in the vicissitude of their search for healing, as painful and challenging as that may have been. I will forever be grateful and remain humbled by the courage and determination they displayed as they faced their demons and ghosts from their past. I also acknowledge my coauthor, Dr. William Herron, who over the years managed to push me into addressing the very issues covered in this and other publications and in the process forcing me to enter a journey of my own to explore difficult moments in that journey of the issues covered in this book. My involvements in the APA-Div 39 Holmes Commission and the CERCCL at the New York University Postdoctoral Program also prompted me to take on a more active role in addressing issues of multisectionality in psychology and particularly in psychoanalytic intervention and training. And then we have others whose contributions may have been indirect and yet still very helpful. I am referring to my administrative assistant, Maureen Robertson, who steadily and reliably managed the affairs of my office and thus gave me the space needed to allow me to focus on the work necessary for the completion of the book. My student Anna Giannicchi should also be acknowledged for her skillful review of some of the material covered in the book.

—Rafael Art. Javier

Introduction

This book describes and promotes the use of integrated psychotherapy as the most effective current mental health delivery system. Advocating this approach is in contrast to most books on psychotherapy because they promote a singular, relatively exclusive method. Their endorsement is based on the alleged value of a particular system due to its apparent effectiveness. Psychoanalysis was a favored approach for some time, with the evidence for effectiveness based primarily on case studies and an appealing philosophy of personality reconstruction. Currently it has been replaced by behavioral approaches where effectiveness is heralded as evidence-based, the evidence being research studies and it has the appeal of relative brevity.

It seems accurate to describe psychoanalysis as being more faith-based and subjectively appealing in its promise of an examined mind, but not providing research studies of its effects, and being lengthy. As a result, its costs and effectiveness clinically became questionable. Behavior therapy has gained ascendancy, supposedly based primarily on its evidence-based research studies. However, the complexity of measuring outcomes and researching psychotherapy ingredients and results indicates the significant limitations of proving value. Based on current knowledge, it is accurate to say that both psychoanalysis and behavior therapy can have value rather than one being exclusively superior to the other. It is likely that the chief appeal of behavioral approaches, including medication, is the shorter duration and in turn cost limitation which fits the current managed-care approach to providing mental health services.

Based on the continued evidence of mental health problems in our society, neither approach has been impressive in dealing with mental illness. At the same time, what can be seen in all approaches is selective effectiveness, which in turn supports the idea of integration as offering a greater probability of improvement for the ineffective system now in place. In essence, use all that we have selectively, custom designed for each patient

In assembling the components for integration, it became apparent that there was an emphasis on either behavioral change or the examined mind, but not on the value of bringing them together. Given that each has value, and can be interconnected, we believe that the use of both, crafted for each patient in terms of frequency and style of use, has the greatest probability of assuring mental health.

Both behavioral methods and psychoanalytic approaches have shown recognition of their need to retrofit to broaden their approaches. The point of any psychotherapy is to help the patient feel and function better, thus the process needs to be patient-centered. Patients deserve the opportunity for self-examination and behavioral change with the understanding that the methods used are in accord with a patient's goals. Psychotherapists' allegiance needs to be to what works for the patient, and that means integrating therapies.

In assembling the material to make our case we found the treatment situation involves understanding the broader social context in which people live, develop culturally, and create self-images and representations of others. Psychotherapy is played out in a complex setting with contradictions, intersectionalities, and interconnections that have a significant impact on our efforts. As a result, there will be repetitive themes in the various chapters that while each has its singular points, these points are designed to elaborate an improved mental health delivery system.

The first chapter describes the current state of mental health treatment with an emphasis on its limitations and the value of integration as a significant attempt at improvement. Although we believe that both behavioral and psychoanalytic approaches need to be retrofitted, our expertise is psychoanalytic, so we provide details for that in the second and third chapters. There has been an emphasis on pluralism which lends support to the viability of psychoanalytic therapies. Also, there has been a detailed examination of the validity of key psychoanalytic concepts which facilitate retrofitting. Our emphasis is on what works for the individual patient, so symptom alleviation and treating a broad spectrum of patients are significant goals of this approach. In each chapter we reiterate a societal and political shift away from the managed care model to improve access to therapy whenever needed and controlled by patient-therapist accord. While aware of the cost involved, we believe this is an issue that needs informed and ongoing advocacy, and that there is no evidence that prior to managed care there were excessive psychotherapy expenses. Unfortunately, the current management method uses difficulties in assessing the needs and results of mental health treatment to allege a need for control; that is a failed and deceptive program.

We realize that our proposed funding alternatives are likely to be in the distant future, but our integrative approach can be applied now. In Chapter 4 we provide several clinical examples of this approach in action. Chapter 5 considers the issue of intersectionality, funding possibilities, and the integrative approach in psychotherapy training with clinical examples, specific integrative issues, possible etiologies of disorders, and repairing the mental health system to serve the type of patients seeking help now. We conclude this chapter with an emphasis on what can be done now via integration. Chapter 6 provides a review of the evidence for the outcome of the psychotherapies. This chapter shows the difficulties involved in evaluation, the relative equivalence of different therapies, the search for therapeutic effects, support for integration, and the need for ongoing research. Chapter 7 probes a specialized issue in treatment, namely the impact that language has in treatment, a contextual assessment that shows there are complex linguistic pathways that require integration as part of the treatment process. Given the increasing presence of patients from a variety of ethnic backgrounds, this is an important issue that has been given limited coverage. Clinical illustrations and findings are provided.

Chapter 8 considers the role of neuroscience in psychotherapeutic exchanges. This chapter combines theoretical and research findings with case examples. Chapter 9 provides an illustration of how psychodynamic and behavioral concepts can be used in the evaluation of patients in forensic contexts. In Chapter 10 we summarize our findings and draw conclusions. We believe there is sufficient evidence that the current mental health delivery system is defective and in need of repair. In broad strokes this means the elimination of restrictive management that is designed to support the health of insurance companies rather than the mental health of all those insured. More immediately, it means integrated treatment in contrast to the prevailing behavioral model and the retrofitting of all the therapies used. Given that the current outlier is psychoanalysis, we describe in detail how that model can be improved, and we indicate, with clinical examples, how integrated, client-centered therapy works.

Mental Health Treatment

Mental health treatment has a disturbing tradition of limited effectiveness. Accurate measurement of treatment results is difficult, though attempts have been made, and research continues. However, existing results support the limitations, and at the moment there are no specific reasons to endorse the belief that what we are doing is that effective. At the same time the incidence of mental illness is increasing, straining a struggling system of mental health providers that function within a complex of personal, social, and economic factors. Treatment is contextual, which adds an element of depersonalization to situations that feel intensely personal to patients. On the positive side, there is a greater awareness and understanding of the elements of mental disorders, and despite the limitations of available treatment, there is an increasing demand for what does exist. The treatment climate for mental disorders has always been unfavorable in innumerable ways, and despite being subjected to many potential remedies, it remains unacceptable. What we are doing just does not work very well, so once again, it is necessary to make some significant changes.

We recognize the complexity of the issue, namely that it goes well beyond coming up with a new specific treatment, so our aim here is modest, incremental improvements through integration and modification of therapeutic possibilities. That does include all modes of available treatment, but our emphasis is on what we know based on our training and experience, which has been psychoanalytic. As a result, we stress modifications in psychoanalytically based treatment procedures.

Particular credit needs to be given to Wachtel (2011) who has been a pioneer in the integration of psychotherapies with his cyclical psychodynamic approach and provides us with jumping-off points.

We also believe that retrofitting, namely continual improvements in all approaches including behavior and pharmaceutical therapies, also needs to be ongoing, but the specifics need to be provided by experts in those areas. We believe no one therapy is effective for all types of mental illness. Instead, we believe that treatment should be patient-specific, essentially varying with the needs of the individual patient. Nothing works all the time with every person, but impressed by human resiliency, we believe there are solutions to some degree for many more people than are getting them. We work from the viewpoint that something can work given that time is taken to make a proper fit for the patient and that the therapist, given appropriate resources, is sufficiently skilled and motivated.

The Modern Treatment Area

The primary background for mental health treatment involved the development of psychoanalysis as talk therapy as well as psychotropic drugs aimed at the alleviation of symptoms, though other treatments existed, such as behavioral therapies and ECT. However, psychoanalysis and drug therapies were revolutionary events, seemed to hold a lot of promise, and got extensive use in some form such as psychoanalytic psychotherapy. A major positive effect of these developments was the removal of a considerable amount of the negative societal attitude toward mental illness. Treatment became more acceptable and in some instances, such as psychoanalysis, relatively popular.

Unfortunately, the enthusiasm did not match the results. Neither medication nor talk therapy made that much of a difference in the overall incidence of mental illness or the apparent recovery from it. There was little research on effectiveness, but enthusiasm for the new treatments led to deinstitutionalization at more than a measured pace. The latter was supposedly aimed at improving the lives of institutionalized patients, with the side effect of reducing costs. However, many patients were not prepared for such a change, and a significant homeless population was created that also disrupted the social order, so the cost to society remained and may well have increased. Behavior therapy overtook psychoanalysis, which had not paid attention to the need for outcome research, and drugs were not nearly as effective as desired in removing symptoms. In essence, mental health treatment became different, more appealing in its apparent brevity and outpatient focus, but it did not become significantly more effective.

Also, in what appeared to be a desired cost saving for consumers, insurance carriers expanded to cover mental health and increased the number of eligible providers. This made treatment more available. However, just as shutting down long-term care facilities fostered the problem of homelessness, insurance created a control shift from the providers of care to the providers of payment, and in turn, restricted care in terms of length and provider choice.

It is difficult to find a balanced account of the various possible approaches for treating mental health because advocates of each plan have understandable preferences for whatever they do themselves. However, Gnaulati (2018) presents a comprehensive view from which it is possible to conclude that medication can be useful rather than curative, that health insurance can be helpful when it is not restrictive, and that talk therapy should be a basic part of the mix. These conclusions support treatment integration but with modifications to existing approaches. For example, employer-sponsored insurance does not do anything for the unemployed, nor does various limitations, such as cost and coverage restrictions do anything for the homeless.

Regarding the homeless and mentally ill, of which there are many, Henninger (2018, p. 15) comments, "Decades ago, progressives pushed the unprecedented social experiment known as deinstitutionalization of the severely mentally ill. Hospital beds were never replaced. Promised off-site care eroded. It is a massive policy failure, with many of the abandoned, mostly male patients, destructively self-medicating on the streets with alcohol and heroin. The chance of reversing this . . . experiment is about zero."

That comment is from a conservative author and has inaccuracies. The experiment did not start in this country, and we believe it was well-intended but not effective. Hospital beds took their hospitals and long-term care with them. Most important, recovery does have to happen. Ways must be found to have this happen.

Current Mental Health Delivery

At present the provision of therapeutic health services is especially dependent on third party payers, whether private insurers, such as United Health Care, or public, such as Medicare. Patients without any insurance support are in the minority. As a result, it is not unusual for patients to have as their first question to a potential therapist, "Are you in my plan?" Although the question is understandable, therapists would prefer the initial question to be about their competence. Patients may assume that the insurance companies are somehow guaranteeing the providers' effectiveness, but they are not. While providers are required to have basic credentials, such as a license to practice, the main attraction for the payers is the willingness of the providers to accept the conditions of employment rather than detailed evidence of providers' skills. So, for patients, the chances of getting the most effective providers are reduced before starting therapy due to the reliance on insurance plans. Instead of choosing therapists based on perceived skills, patients get a limited menu. Not only are payers setting fees but they also restrict the number of providers available to patients. From the payers' point of view, this is ideal cost control, but it is not an ideal therapeutic service for patients. However, the argument can be made that if providers set the fee, they would exclude a significant number of people who could not afford the services so that the "good-enough" therapy now provided is really the best arrangement for most people. It is certainly an open question as to how therapists would deal with the economic issue, but it is likely that in the current marketplace, some patients would be priced out because they have insurance coverage.

The reality for all health services is that the cost requires a subsidy to meet the standard of living that is deemed appropriate by providers and that the standard of living is relatively "in place" to keep attracting providers for essential services such as health. The appropriate issue then is how to provide the best quality care at an acceptable level for both payers and providers, and the current answer, managed care that is controlled by neither patients nor providers is inadequate.

Certainly, this is a complex issue that involves the greater good of society, which of course is defined in different ways by the different segments of the society. A consensus could consist of a sufficient number of people that feel they are satisfied with the way health services are provided, but the ongoing push to expand affordable services indicates that the consensus is not in place. Our concern is psychotherapy, and for that service to be at its most effective it means that both patients and therapists have to be satisfied with the way the services are provided. If in all cases patients could seek out whatever therapist they wanted, it is unlikely that patients and therapists would agree often enough on the cost issue to meet the actual need, given that the majority of serious mental health problems are being treated in public facilities where fees are subsidized, and treatment is less than optimal. In private practice, even using a sliding scale requires enough patients at the high end to balance the low end, essentially limiting how many low-end patients would be included; yet that is the larger group in need.

The demographics of mental health needs cannot be met without an external support system, which provided the opportunity for the creation of employer-sponsored health benefits. This has become the norm for all health services, but the control of how the services are sponsored went to the sponsors and away from providers and patients. This situation was acceptable to those being serviced as long as they believed they were getting good quality care, and it was acceptable to the providers as long as they felt they were being compensated appropriately. However, there have been tipping points that resulted in a focus on cost containment rather than quality of care. In practice what had appeared reasonable got reshaped into lower payments for providers and limited care. The prevailing approach has become rapid, least expensive, symptomatic care that is less than satisfying to both patients and providers.

Treatment for mental illness has been an easy target for manipulation because the effects of the available therapies are so difficult to evaluate. Research has usually been limited in scope and sophistication. Also, the various therapies have emphasized their individual values as most worthwhile and marginalized other possibilities. The "evidence-based" phrase needs to be revised to "evidence-biased." The reality is that what appears to work some of the time, also fails, and that we need everything that can work selected based on each patient's needs. Unfortunately, at present, treatment at public facilities that see a larger number of patients is a revolving door. There are no long-term affordable inpatient facilities. Outpatient treatment is medication and behavior therapy, without hard evidence of effectiveness, is time-limited. The result is that psychotherapists have some new shoes to walk in that do not cover enough distance for their patients. Time keeps proving the ongoing, lengthy complications of mental illness. There is a pressing need to make changes in the way we are doing things.

We have several suggestions, the first being that as therapists we need to be strong advocates for providing effective services. To advocate we must provide evidence of effectiveness that goes beyond belief in what we already doing to illustrate that patients improve as a result of what we are doing. This evidence requires examination of case material on a clinical level and controlled studies that include long-term therapies. Gathering evidence means continually being alert for understanding psychopathology and considering ways to mitigate or eliminate it. There has been excessive faith in what we do based on specific theoretical beliefs involved in our training. We have to keep examining what we do and keep considering how it can be improved.

Also, observing the flow of anxiety in each patient, and in the environment in which we live, strongly supports the long-lasting nature of mental illness, which in turn means that a healthy society needs greater access to treatment than is currently available. Weinberger and Stoycheva (2020) state "successful therapy is likely to take time, effortful repetition, and continuous monitoring . . . effective therapy is long-term therapy, and/or interventions that are repeated periodically" (p. 318).

Funders need to focus more on helping people feel better more of the time rather than cost reduction, and as therapists, we have to keep advocating for that focus. We have too long tried to stay above the fray, to be apolitical, only to be continually limited and restricted in what we do. The need for a good patient-therapist fit requires access to a wider range of providers and therapies that are now made available based on financial support. For example, if private insurers were to follow the lead of Traditional Medicare and not have such restrictive networks, then that would be a major improvement. Contrast Medicare Advantage (a private insurance often masquerading as Traditional Medicare) with Traditional Medicare. The former is a network of Medicare providers chosen by private insurers, so it limits the number of possible providers, while the latter offers services from all Medicare providers. The supposed advantage is that some services are not covered by Traditional Medicare but are covered by Medicare Advantage. However, as we write this, Congress is attempting to provide the missing coverage. Is it an advantage to lose the choice of providers for services that may not be used? Perhaps, if the services do get used, the proposed extension of Traditional Medicare is a better option.

From therapists' viewpoints, capped fees, such as Medicare, are not ideal, but if the fees are fair, which at the moment is debatable, then access is what really matters for the health of society. However, a negotiated fee between therapist and patient was traditionally a component of the process that began a familiar duality of control, so it would be more comfortable for therapists, but patients seem to like the cap because it seems to remove their economic concern. Although they pay for insurance, it seems as if the cost issue is settled in advance. It is not that much of an adjustment for therapists and creates certainty for them regarding payment. The probability now is that health insurance in some form will be the usual payment process for therapy. The troubling issue is that it is linked to other aspects of the therapy, such as coverage by diagnostic category, session length, and duration of therapy, which are linked to progress and more effectively controlled by patient-therapist agreement.

The economic factor does have to be considered as it remains a significant factor in therapy, regardless of its source. A possible compromise for payers, therapists, and patients could be that there would be a designated yearly amount for mental health via insurance that would provide a significant percentage of a generally agreed-upon fee considered in total to be adequate and fair by all concerned. That amount would be adequate to cover at least a year of once-a-week sessions. Such an approach would allow for therapist-patient control of the per-session fee while providing an insured floor for patients. This is one possibility, and others could be advanced that are viable. The point is, payment requires significant consideration in planning mental health delivery.

The fact that we are making a suggestion regarding payment, and inviting others, indicates the degree to which control of basic parameters of traditional psychotherapy has moved from therapist-patient control to third-party control. The situation presents a serious obstacle to designing the optimal patient-therapist model including the ingredients of therapists' qualifications, duration, frequency, and length of sessions, and, of course, payment for services. Currently, patients will most often go to therapists designated by their insurance companies and therapists will be part of a network created by the payers. That network adheres to rules for the treatment that includes duration, fee, frequency of treatment, and diagnostic categories that will be covered. The treatment is not individualized to a significant extent, other than by limitations, and it is not designed by the participants in the treatment.

Although the participants are relatively unlimited in what they can say to each other, various aspects of the therapy may have to be revealed to justify the progress of the therapy to the payers, thus limiting confidentiality beyond what is customary for the protection of self and others. The treatment will usually consist of brief behavioral techniques. In public settings this will usually be accompanied by medication. The emphasis is on cost containment, not treatment quality. Gnaulati (2018) refers to this type of treatment as "managed care-lessness" (p. 90), which is painfully accurate. There is an irony in the current situation in that when insurance first began covering mental health treatment, they allowed clinical considerations to be made by practitioners. However, there was a lack of understanding of the complexity of mental disorders and mental health treatment. It takes an undetermined amount of time to provide psychotherapy properly in each case, and it is difficult to quantify results given the subjectivity involved. As a result, psychotherapy was an easy target for utilization review that could support a need to "manage" care. Curtailment became inevitable, and so has the decline in the quality of care. The lack of understanding continues in the recent "No Surprises" act where the cost and length of treatment are potentially to be applied to psychotherapy before treatment.

Psychotherapists need to develop a powerful voice for open access (no networks) and open duration for psychotherapy. As Weinberger and Stoycheva (2020) note, "it is not impossible to alter maladaptive behaviors, affective reactions, and habits of thought, but it is not easy either" (p. 318). They point out that relapses are frequent and it takes a long time before the positive effects can be maintained. Of course, for therapy to be effective, current costs will increase, but the cost of a relatively unlimited approach is offset by the potential increase of people in therapy who will indeed require less other medical treatment. In addition, it would be a minor increase in the overall health bill. Unlimited access to psychotherapy would not result in an overwhelming use because a major problem with mental health treatment has always been, and will remain, getting people to use it, and if they do, remain in it long enough to realize the benefits. Still, making it more available increases the chances of greater usage.

The rumblings about Medicare for all are hopeful, provided that such a policy avoids an emphasis on management. Therapists must foster an awareness that quality mental health treatment is a political issue in which we have a large stake, so they cannot stay on the sideline while legislation is drafted and enacted. As a large group of providers, we have been too quiet about the creation, continued presence, and growth of these excluding, arbitrary networks that are essentially small monopolies designed to benefit their creators rather than help patients. Regardless of theoretical orientations, patient needs should be the voice of practice. Thus, we go on record for open-access psychotherapy for whatever patients need for as long as it is needed. Whatever it costs would be a small price to pay for the potential improvement of the mental health of society.

We also have been too quiet about other issues involved in providing mental health services. De-institutionalization is not an effective replacement for long-term care facilities. Many patients cannot function effectively outside of the structured environments that had been provided by mental hospitals. While it is a good idea to also provide less structured treatment environments, that does not mean the more structured ones should be eliminated, or exist solely for patients who can afford to pay for their care. Hospitals need to be replaced and improved, rather than removed.

Assumptions that mental disorders, particularly psychoses, for certain have genetic or biological etiologies are not established facts. We do not know what causes mental disorders. We only know what factors appear to contribute to their presence, and the most likely explanation is a mixture of factors, such as a diathesis-stress theory. Neuroscience is helpful in identifying areas of brain functioning that may be involved, but it is not identifying etiology, the latter remaining relatively mysterious and frequently seemingly individualized. Official diagnostic systems, as DSM and ICD are supposed attempts at evidence-based diagnoses that focus on observable behavior, but neglect overall personality functioning. Although that has not gone unnoticed, the psychodynamic diagnostic manual (PDM-2) (Lingardi & McWilliams, 2017) is unfortunately not a practical answer. The diagnosis of mental disorders usually has to be made rapidly to facilitate treatment. While sympathetic to the philosophy of the PDM, namely diagnosis as a combination of an individual's external and internal experiences, such an understanding is usually apparent only through lengthy observation. Most of the time there is not a sufficient duration for treatment planning that would meet the PDM criteria. We suggest the PDM once again be refined, but actually "simplified," to take it beyond interesting and into the area of practical widespread usage.

The Next Step

Although there are certainly flaws in the current mental health delivery system, there have also been positive developments. Awareness and acceptance of mental health issues have increased significantly. More people are open to recognizing mental health issues in themselves and others. There is greater demand for, and usage of, mental health services. The importance of mental health for society is gaining parity with physical health, and the mind-body connection has gained considerable recognition. Within the field of mental health services, the continuing development of psychotropic medications is a major assist for treatment protocols. There has been an increase in the treatment possibilities that are available to consumers, and most insurance plans now provide coverage for mental disorders.

At the same time, increased demand for services does require more providers, and that has loosened the standards of providers' skill sets. The majority of patients receive services in public institutions where the providers often have the least amount of training. Rosenberg (2018) reports that almost half of the adult population in this country utilizes mental health services, and the number is similar for children and adolescents. Most of the patients are being treated by master's level clinicians, and the number of these providers is twice the size of doctoral level clinicians (psychologist, psychiatrist).

Without disparaging the efforts made by clinicians with limited training, it remains clear that the majority of patients are being treated by therapists who are the least equipped to treat them. This situation is a result of several factors. The increase in demand for services has not been matched by an increase in funding for more extensive training. Instead, costs are being offset by hiring less skilled workers. Accompanying this trend is the theory that the combination of drug application and brief behavioral therapy can provide satisfactory outcomes. The reality is that current restrictive approaches are a recipe for continuing illness.

Psychoanalysis and its relatives, psychoanalytic and psychodynamic therapies, have been victims of such managed care. They are being excluded from the roster of treatment possibilities because they are considered too lengthy, in turn, too expensive, and not that effective to be worth considering. Psychoanalytic approaches have been replaced by behavioral treatments that are short term, and less expensive, and have been put forth as "evidence-based." Medication is also routine. However, mental health delivery and treatment remain ineffective.

What has this new era of care brought us then, beyond marginalizing psychoanalysis? We have noted the increased awareness of mental health problems and the acceptance of the need for treatment, but the increased demand brought increased costs that were considered unacceptable. The lack of cost acceptance resulted in managed care which claimed to provide effective treatment that would be brief and relatively inexpensive. In essence mental illness was put in a disease category that could be "cured," along with the idea that this could happen quickly (and, perhaps, permanently). Mental illness has always been misunderstood. Any classification of it has inadequacies, although there is a practical need to categorize and treat it. Left untreated, meaning without organized, systematized efforts to alleviate it, the damage to individuals and society would be unacceptable. However, in the mix of capitalism and humanitarianism that has been our culture, the emphasis has been on cost reduction rather than quality of care.

The existing methodology is ineffective. Mental illness cannot be cured, that is removed in the fashion of an offending appendix. Mental health is a lifelong issue that varies for everyone, depending on genetics and environment. It affects mind and body, behavior, thought, and affect. The most common symptoms, anxiety and depression, are felt to some degree by everybody at different times in their lives. The more extreme forms, such as disordered thinking and anti-social behavior, are tendencies of the human condition. The illness category comes into play when functioning becomes impaired and gets specified based on symptoms, as a symptom cluster such as schizophrenia, or a pervasive symptom, such as persistent anxiety.

There are no treatment strategies that work all of the time or for every illness. A realistic aim is the mitigation of pathology and sufficient functionality for a person to lead an acceptable life. The movement from unacceptable to acceptable behavior patterns is a stacking procedure, new on top of old, where new dominates but old remains in circulation, rather than a removal-replacement operation. Maladaptive patterns can and do return, depending on situational factors. Thus, our emphasis is on open-access treatment possibilities. Also varying with individuals is the length of any treatment, so, again, the value in eliminating treatment duration limits.

While it is markedly difficult to get "true" measures of therapeutic progress, and etiologies remain hypothetical, there is sufficient evidence that most of the existing therapies have value for different individuals. This suggests that therapeutic integration is a more effective path to pursue than making one therapeutic protocol standard and disregarding others, which has been the prevailing tendency.

Effective mental health treatment does require eliminating several bad ideas. The first is the management of treatment by people outside the patient-therapist mix. People seek therapy out of a need and continue in therapy to alleviate problems that tend to be painful and persistent. Until these are sufficiently mitigated the treatment needs to continue, meaning it should be open-ended. Why not?

Because there will be unnecessary treatment. Why assume this? Both patients and therapists are seeking success, which translates into patients feeling good enough to get along without therapy and therapists feeling pleased with that result. Patients also save money and gain time for other pursuits if they have completed therapy, and if their situation becomes problematic again, they can return. As for therapists, there are more than enough patients to keep them busy, so it is not an economic issue.

Also, provider panels need to go. The "fit" between therapist and patient has often been found as a major factor in patient improvement. There needs to be "open access" to providers based on the choice of the therapy participants, not on the designation of an insurer. The licensing procedures already in place can serve as the guardians of competence and can be revised accordingly if there are failures to do so. The disciplines involved in treatment need to keep developing progress measurements that meet standards of reliability and validity, publish the results, and keep both training facilities and the public aware of probable effectiveness. Current management arrangements assume devious motivations by both therapists and patients, restrict the effectiveness of treatment, and primarily benefit the managers, which is not supposed to be the purpose of the management.

Drug therapy is useful, but limited by some factors such as side effects, compliance resistance, variable success rates, and it appears to work most effectively when combined with talk therapy, which unfortunately is usually being "managed" with the aim of cost control. In that context the therapies being offered are usually behavioral, despite these methods having no greater effectiveness than psychodynamic methods. The effects of the drugs do require significant compliance, so there is an ongoing problem of under-use (I do not want to be dependent on drugs) or over-use (I need more than is being given). The medications are aimed at symptom reduction, with the idea of gradually moving the patient off their usage rather than it being a lifetime procedure. However, some patients tend to rely solely on the drug, which is convenient but activates the probability of addiction or side effects, such as insomnia and weight gain, which can result in other problems.

If the problems that we described, primarily the managed-care, cost-reduction, this-is really-good-enough approach could be eliminated, that would be a great start to improving service delivery. The existing research indicates the effectiveness of a pluralistic approach to treatment. This means the integration of treatments, and in particular, the reclamation of psychodynamic methods that have been marginalized by the existing behavioral philosophy of treatment. The current approach appears to be a form of restraint of trade, although patients can see any provider they desired, provided they can pay for it. Given that cost, a large number of patients could not afford to make that choice, so they remain in the network. The "forced" aspect of this procedure is covered by the assertion that the providers are of high quality, and so is the treatment. But then why not let patients have choices? We see the idea that removing current management would result in an excessive cost as deceptive. At this time, we are in the midst of a mental health crisis as part of the viral spread that has upended all our lives. Society in general approves spending money to alleviate it, with benefits outweighing costs. With growing awareness of the importance of mental health, it should be clear that making it affordable to all is a priority. We already have programs, such as Social Security, Medicare, and Medicaid that are major steps to ensuring the overall health of the society. These programs are elastic in that they provide flexibility to expand coverage and could be used to replace current restrictions that are designed in such a way that mental health treatment is constricted.

Ironically, Gnaulati (2018) points out that until 1973 when the Health Maintenance Organization Act was signed into law, insurance coverage was widely available for mental health services. Therapists and patients determined the type and amount of psychotherapy, therapist choice was not restricted, and insurers were billed directly. Fees were paid as long as they were considered reasonable, with patients often having a modest copay. The situation was altered by raising the specter of possible excessive health costs without a more stringent utilization review. We have already noted the difficulty in assessing accurately the results of psychotherapy, and in addition, the therapy field did not present a united front regarding treatment issues, such as frequency and duration. Claiming to provide better for less, managed care came in. The result has been the reduction of quality as provider panels were formed based on participants' acceptance of insurance-determined fees rather than competence. Psychotherapy was an easy target as provider fees decreased, but insurers' profits increased. The fact that a working system had been in place was ignored. The promised quality care is now often careless, a trend very much in need of being reversed. There are seeds of hope, such as Obamacare and the proposed Medicare for all, but little agreement on how to improve the overall health system, which, in terms of cost, mental health is a minor player.

There is no evidence to support the belief that the type of unfettered mental health care that we are proposing would be an excessive cost for the national health budget. People do not choose mental health services based primarily on cost but on need and a belief that some relief can be found by using them. In that regard, people have always been wary of using such services, so the possibility of their availability at low or moderate cost is not going to create an influx of consumers. Paris (2013) points out that only about 3% of Americans begin psychotherapy, and that half of them drop out after the second visit. As already noted, mental health treatment has never had an attractive reputation, which is all the more a reason to reform rather than restrict coverage. Gnaulati (2018) points out that the public policy issue is that so many people fail to use psychotherapy that it is difficult to even approach meaningful progress. We need to do better, and we can afford to make the attempt. Our issue here is how to improve.

As psychoanalytic psychotherapists, we operate in a broad social context where we are both influencers and are influenced. To indicate accurately what we can do we believe it has been necessary to begin by illustrating in some detail the broad social field in which we work. In so doing we have shown the existing problems in delivering mental health services and have suggested significant changes. However, the main thrust of this book is to show how our specialty, the psychoanalytic approach, deserves to be used as a major agent of change. This represents a significant alteration from the current marginalization of psychoanalytic approaches that deprives patients of significant opportunities for improving their lives. For our enterprise to be successful, we propose the retrofitting of psychoanalysis.

Integrated Psychotherapy

To retrofit means to change what exists to create improvement, namely, make a better model. The focus in psychotherapy has to be on the outcome. We operate to make people feel better, to function better, and to be better people, and we have a process to do that. The process needs continued evaluations in terms of the goal, and psychoanalysis has always recognized such a need. At the same time, it has been selective and exclusionary rather than seeking to always incorporate what works and leave what does not work. The goal has often been more influenced by the therapist's aims than by what the patient wanted. Analysts aimed at patients having an "analysis," based on the belief that value for the patient was created by having an examined mind. Such a mind was considered to logically make the patient feel better, and in turn, act better. Unfortunately, such an approach did not necessarily remove symptoms, make the patient feel better, or act better, though it was likely to improve the patient's personal understanding. Also, sometimes it did some or all of the other desired alterations, but it was lengthy, costly, and resistive to the resistant, meaning patients who wanted something more practical and immediate. It is fair to say that psychoanalysis seemed effective in making people feel different but stumbled in facilitating the transfer of that difference into functional improvement. Of course, over time changes have been made in service of improving theory, method, and possible results, for example, instinctual gave way to relational and orthodoxy to pluralism, but integration with other approaches was suspect and limited. Evidence of success was more a matter of faith than detailed measurement.

The complexity of the issue is a major difficulty in assessing the value of any mental health treatment. The patient is the final judge, but the patient's judgment is suspect, as is the therapist's opinion, because of the high degree of subjectivity involved. More objective criteria do exist but are limited in scope as descriptions of individual mental states. There is the presence of resistance to change that always appears even though there may be an acknowledgement of both the need to change as well as desire. Etiology is uncertain, hypothetical, and far from universal. Any claim that one therapy is better than another because one is "evidence-based" is tenuous at best. The evidence requires examination and awareness of its limited reliability and validity (Wachtel, 2010).

Nonetheless, it remains essential that evidence-gathering continues and that therapists learn about what seem to be promising therapeutic methods. Of course, the fact remains that patients' subjectivity contributes to therapists' distrust of outcome research, as well as its known limitations.

Case studies are also useful, but subject to a variety of opinions. There are some more objective indicators, such as mood and behavioral shifts. However, despite limitations, therapists are there to satisfy patients and symptom alleviation is usually foremost with patients. Behavioral approaches have capitalized on this, so it is important to factor in when considering integrative approaches.

To retrofit it is necessary to look at all the elements of the process to see how they contribute to the outcome. Psychoanalytic theory is distinguished by the most extensive and comprehensive system designed to describe behavior and promote change. The scope of the theory is daunting, but recently Eagle (2018a, 2018b) published two volumes, *Core Concepts in Classical Psychoanalysis* and *Core Concepts in Contemporary Psychoanalysis*, which examine the research into basic psychoanalytic concepts that have been central to the ongoing practice of psychoanalysis. For classical psychoanalysis, he considered unconscious processes, the Oedipus complex, inner conflict, and defense. For contemporary psychoanalysis, he focused on transference and countertransference as well as discussing projective identification.

These volumes are a major contribution to the evaluation of psychoanalytic theory. They demonstrate the variety of meanings attached to the different constructs as well as the validity of the constructs. Since treatment is based on theory, such data is particularly helpful in providing pathways for effective therapy. In essence he provides evidence for what works as well as what does not work. A major conclusion is that there is strong evidence that psychoanalysis can use a major retrofit. While the books do not attempt to encompass the entire theory, they certainly do cover key concepts. As such they are very helpful in determining needed alterations that in turn could lead to empirical outcomes.

The existence of the unconscious, a basic concept for all psychoanalytic approaches, is well supported. However, the role of the unconscious, including its contents and role influencing behavior, remains open to investigation. A large part of mental life exists outside of awareness and is influenced by unconscious factors, so people often behave for reasons of which they are unaware, but there is not substantial evidence that it is the emotional nature of the motivation, for example, unacceptable sexual desires, that results in the lack of awareness. Nonetheless, the concept of repression may well exist, but repression would be a broad concept. Instead of mental content being repressed, meaning kept out of consciousness because of its disturbing effect, it could be because of what we term "more mundane" reasons, as it happened too long ago to remember. At the same time, it could influence behavior as unaware learning. Given the increasing amount of unconscious experience relative to conscious life, it is very difficult to establish specific links between unconscious motivations and psychopathology. The unconscious appears to be dynamic, but more incidental than weighty in influencing behavior.

As for Oedipus, it is indeed a myth. It can occur, but it is one of many relational outcomes that appear as individuals develop an identity, a self as distinct from being part of another. The triangular Oedipal situation serves as a limited description of a possible pathway to gender identity, but it is simplistic, based on the possible primacy of sexual motivation and its involvement in the development of psychopathology. Sexual desire is an important motivation, but only one of many. Lichtenberg (1989) made that point some time ago, but it had a limited impact. Eagle reiterates it, mentioning aggression, attachment, self-regulation, and caregiving as other possibilities. He also notes the importance of interaction among motivational systems rather than the reduction of systems to a superordinate one. The evidence suggests that there is individual variability among interactive motivational systems that results in specific motivational hierarchies. The outcome of identity formation, object seeking, and superego development, as well as their motivations, rest on the interactive complexities of varying genetic, social, and environmental developmental forces.

Conflict has always been a central feature of psychoanalytic understanding. As a result, there are numerous descriptions of inner conflict as well as theories connected to them, with an ongoing search for "fundamental" conflicts. In that respect, there has been a shift in emphasis from early developmental conflicts about sexual and aggressive desires to desires for autonomy and individuation. This shift expands the view of conflict origination and stresses the influence of the developmental environment. Other shifts include guilt as well as anxiety being prominent in conflict, symbolic equivalence, and the importance of the ability to both delay and experience gratification.

Eagle also points out that despite the frequent emphasis on inner conflict, originally linked to sex and aggression, there is a turn toward the idea of deficits. Although both deficit and conflict models are both active, psychopathology can be understood in terms of maladaptive representations. Evidence supports a broad view of the causes of psychopathology as being deficiencies in ego functioning. Interpretations that lead to greater self-understanding serve to support ego functioning, though other factors, as reflective capacity and intersubjectivity, are also important. Basically, there is movement toward a pluralistic, expansive understanding of possible etiological factors. The support for the influence of unconscious motivation includes the concept of defense as a necessary component of functioning.

Cramer (2006, 2008) provides a detailed description of defenses at work protecting the self, relationalities, and diminishing negative emotions. However, Eagle points out that people are not as unaware of their defensive maneuvers as had been assumed. Instead, the role of the preconscious has to be reconsidered as relatively active with more recognition given to the level of self-awareness. Also, the context of each person's situation requires consideration in regard to the value of defense analysis. In essence, therapeutic success will rest on varying degrees of self-knowledge.

In terms of retrofitting, the quality of the unconscious requires expansion to give more room to the degree of probable personal awareness and the content of the material. In particular, some representations are acquired earlier in life and reinforced by the potential for conflict with disturbing effects, such as anxiety and depression. While infantile wishes may be present regarding sex and aggression, separation and individuation concerns appear significant, if not prominent. It appears that conflicted issues are not articulated, or formulated, to the degree that they are resolved, but are at some level of awareness. So, knowing yourself is important, but the uncovering of specifics appears less valuable compared to intersubjectivity, individuation, and affect regulation.

Transference and countertransference also require modification. Transference is best defined as the attribution of characteristics of significant others to the therapist. The significant others usually include parents, but it does not have to include them or be restricted to them. Transference of attributes exists in all interpersonal situations based on the anticipation of the situation and the actual behavior of the participants. Some patient reactions are based on projection, meaning unwarranted based on the therapist's behavior, while others are based on the therapist's behavior.

As a result, therapist neutrality is a relative concept. If experienced by the patient as a negative reaction to the patient's needs, it can have a negative influence on the outcome. The context of the situation, the "field of interaction," is the main determiner of what works, and it varies with each patient. Although transference always occurs, there is no evidence that it has to be analyzed, or even investigated, or that it is related to a positive outcome. However, the representation of significant others certainly influences both perceptions of new people and of the self. It is a key component of dynamic relationships between self and object representations and interactional patterns. Transference and countertransference are both intrapsychic and interactional.

Countertransference, the therapist's feelings about the patient, is also based on previous object representations as well as current reactions of the patient and the therapist. It can serve as a useful guide in understanding and responding to patients and is an affective occurrence in the process, but there is no convincing evidence that it is a reliable opening to patients' unconscious. Therapists react emotionally to their patients and these reactions can be useful in understanding patients, but more in the direction of the value of the relationship than in the value of interpretation.

The case for retrofitting is a strong one. Basic psychoanalytic concepts, such as the unconscious, conflict, and transference are well supported by research evidence but require broader definitions and applications. Other conceptions, such as a universal Oedipal complex as the determiner of identity, or the equating of normal developmental stages with adult pathology, have little support. The idea of integration with other approaches, such as behavioral is usually disregarded (by the other approaches as well). From both a practical and theoretical point of view, this attitude needs to be changed. Eagle has provided an excellent reconsideration of some essential psychoanalytic conceptions and has indicated the shift in direction taken by contemporary psychoanalysts. This change is a broadening of conceptions from an emphasis on early and instinctual origins to a greater awareness of multiple motivations at different developmental levels as well as the importance of the therapeutic relationship. This supports further examination of psychoanalytic conceptions and approaches, such as free association, resistance, and suggestion, as well as the need to consider the use of focused and behavioral approaches. In essence, the psychoanalytic approach needs to be relevant by customizing its methodology to the needs and capabilities of patients.

It is probable that from the outset there was an unofficial variability in the clinical application of psychoanalysis. Even Freud would have a stated approach while doing something contradictory. However, it was not until the presence of the relational movement that theoretical differences accompanied by clinical variations gained status as "psychoanalytic." The evidence synthesized by Eagle provides reasons to support developing alterations in theory and practice. Before illustrating our attempts to customize the psychoanalytic approach to make it patient-centered, we will use the next two chapters to illustrate the clinical value of restoring psychoanalytic approaches to the standard therapeutic routines as well as indicating how pluralism is employed in the process.

2

The Clinical Value of Psychoanalysis

The times, they are a'changin'. They have changed. We are writing this as the coronavirus is at the heart of a pandemic altering the way life is for everyone. There is a new layer of anxiety and depression, the effects of which are just beginning to show. The need for mental health treatment, already significant, is increasing, and highlights a notable issue, namely the relevance of psychoanalysis. The unexpected events of a few weeks ago are creating new treatment environments. Our ethical view as providers commits us to work at making available a continually improving service shaped to the shifting needs of patients. This means evolution and alteration of what we are doing intending to make more people feel better. The existing environment is not ideal to do this, but we need to adapt to these new realities as they appear. This is true for all psychotherapists, regardless of one's comfort zone, but the specifics of orientations and traditions complicate this to varying degrees. It is particularly true for those of us trained as psychoanalysts and invested in what has served as the foundation for all psychotherapies.

For some time now psychoanalysts have recognized that to be most effective it was necessary to be continually in the process of retrofitting so that descriptions of what we do now, or propose for the future, is a work in progress. Retrofitting involves making changes to an original model necessitated by new knowledge. This has been the stated mode of psychoanalytic evolution beginning with Freud, and throughout has involved more than one view of the same issue. Gediman (2018) notes that Freud acknowledged that any psychical process can be depicted from varying viewpoints. Perhaps it was a reluctant admission, as retrofitting usually moved slowly and within a limited range, but the idea was always alive. The psychoanalysts who followed Freud chronologically continued with modifications, for example, ego psychology, but a relative orthodoxy prevailed for some time and limited the scope of changes. For many decades it was not possible to stray any distance from Freudian constructs, such as drive theory, and still be considered a psychoanalyst. Dissenters paid the price of marginalization, such as Alexander Horney, among others. Evolution existed as a muted adaptation. Hartmann (1958) introduced the concept of adaptation to psychoanalysis, describing it as a relationship between specific entities, namely the self and the environment, in which the self develops the ability to change both self and/or the environment. Adaptation is a reciprocal relationship, an interactive field of person and surround, both operating as potential agents of change. For some time that concept slanted in favor of the influence of psychoanalysis, which became the treatment of choice as well as a philosophy and culture within the greater society. For many years it appeared as if it indeed might become a psychoanalytic world, until it did not. Now it is not, its influence limited, its validity questioned, its adherents depicted as niche players.

What happened? Adaptation it turns out had not been reciprocal in a sufficient manner. Disruptions came from the internal environment of analysis, and now they came with significant force not only to be heard by analysts but also to be embraced as psychoanalytic. The customary expected adherents failed to materialize. The environment moved against psychoanalysis and instead embraced other treatments as apparently more valid and effective. Potential extinction became a possibility and eradication has been suggested, but that has not happened. A relatively strong psychoanalytic base continues to exist, but psychoanalysis was reshaped and continues to be characterized by diversity rather than orthodoxy. This is a development with mixed features. It is overdue and refreshing in giving voice to new ideas as well as developing standards of accountability for its practices. Also the multitude of voices fosters confusion and can seem chaotic. Particularly vexing is the difficulty in defining psychoanalysis and the increased difficulty in establishing a comprehensive theory with practical guidelines for providing analysis. This has always been a task gone wanting, and it remains that way.

The presence of a comprehensive theory is a pertinent issue for the practice of any psychotherapy because providers should be able to explain to their patients their specific procedures and treatment goals. It is appropriate for patients to expect a relatively unitary description, namely, this is what analysis involves and this is what it aims to accomplish. Instead, the current reality is relatively diverse offerings with rather amorphous aims, all under the psychoanalytic banner, but emphasizing different issues, as instinctual or environmental motivations, and deficit or conflict models of psychopathology. Given that analysis is a product being marketed by its adherents as a treatment for mental disorders, integration would facilitate its presentation.

However, some factors have made integration an elusive possibility. One is the complexity of the therapeutic process itself which is difficult to explain or to quantify. Another is the desire on the part of these many varying schools of thought to be the sole authorized representative of psychoanalysis while debunking the others. Also, this diversity and struggle for distinctive acknowledgment are happening at a time when there has been a marked diminution in the influence of psychoanalysis on both training and provision for mental health services, thereby limiting the potential value of struggling no less winning the struggle. The general societal view appears to have shifted from belief and optimism to doubt and pessimism as to the accuracy and healing power of psychoanalysis.

"Increased *accountability* is especially critical for progress in psychoanalysis because the profession has suffered in the public's eyes due to its sometimes extravagant claims, and it has been weakened by a reliance on faith and dogma as well as an unwillingness to acknowledge shortcomings and mistakes" (Axelrod et al., 2018, p. 273).

Distinctions

As psychotherapies other than psychoanalysis have gained significant acceptance at the expense of psychoanalysis, it remains true that all appear essentially based on some aspect of the original psychoanalytic platform, but this customarily goes unacknowledged by the proponents of these supposedly nonanalytic therapies. This is a disingenuous omission, as Jaffe (2014) points out that "all psychotherapies rely on the same modes of therapeutic action that Freud pioneered a century ago" (p. 8).

The elements of talk therapy used today have been active for some time, beginning with the development of psychoanalysis. It is difficult to be precise as to all the categories of therapeutic action, but Jaffe (2014) has proposed a list that appears appropriately inclusive, and all were used by Freud as he was on his way to developing psychoanalysis. The neglect of accurate origination by nonanalytic therapies is customarily managed through distancing techniques, now that analysis has declined in popularity. The therapy is given a distinctive name accompanied by emphasizing that it lacks any connection to psychoanalysis. This is designed to avoid possible difficulties in adhering to the psychoanalytic model. These therapies represent "psychoanalysis denied."

A different approach is taking place within the psychoanalytic community. This involves developing "new models," meaning these models in some fashion are to be differentiated from the original model. However, they are considered to fit under the psychoanalytic umbrella with implications that they represent a much-needed improvement. These models represent "psychoanalysis repaired." The most radical of these would be a "new psychoanalysis" which represents significant basic changes in the original model. The result of all these alterations is the widespread existence of pluralism in psychoanalysis. We will discuss the impact of pluralism in the next chapter. It is testimony to the need for the evolution of psychoanalysis as an effective treatment model (Jurist, 2018).

Unfortunately, the major contribution of talk therapies to treatment has now moved outside of psychoanalysis and limits the use of psychoanalytic procedures. Cognitive-behavior therapies (CBT) have become the major procedure, accompanied by drug therapy. Psychiatry dominates the procedural rules for mental health treatment, particularly in hospitals and clinics where the majority of patients are, and medication dominates, generally accompanied by CBT. The talk-therapy accompaniment is due to an awareness of the limitations of medication, as side effects, symptomatic focus, and sporadic effectiveness as well as ineffectiveness. Thus, the accompanying talk therapy emphasizes support and coping skills, but with limited attention to structural change or extensive improvement. Talk therapy is certainly used, and considered useful, but limited. Psychoanalysis is considered impractical and ineffective. Insurance coverage often is the ultimate determinant of the type and length of treatment, and emphasis is on cost containment. However, this is not even close to a picture of improved mental health, and there is no evidence to support the "revolving door" of present-day treatment as being effective.

A definitive answer is yet to be found, but the possibility exists of making better use of what is available. There are many mental health treatments, and most of them work some of the time with some people, but there is a lack of conclusive evidence that one form of psychotherapy is better than another. Nonetheless, the possibility exists that the greatest chance of improvement lies in the integration of the components of the different therapies that have demonstrated some significant effectiveness. This translates to the need for developing a significant position for psychoanalysis in treatment protocols. The aim of this book is to illustrate how that can be accomplished.

Given the complexity of the problems that therapists work with, namely the vagaries of human behavior, and the variety of individuals involved, it certainly would be helpful if more definitive "how to" evidence was available, but at present this is certainly not the case. Nonetheless that does not mean there is no suggestive evidence. This will be discussed in a separate chapter, but certain available conclusions are pertinent here as helpful guides. The first is that there is definite support for the effectiveness of talk therapy, but primarily in terms of alleviation of problems rather than their removal (true for medication as well). In addition, therapeutic improvement is most obvious in short-term symptom-targeted therapies. These results are well advertised and have a strong appeal to funding sources, patients, treatment centers, and referral sources based on possible cost, duration, and temporary relief is often enough considered good enough to rule out psychoanalysis as a potential treatment. The fact that it is limited in scope and probable sustainability has not been that significant a reservation, though emotional and practical support for longer-lasting benefits and open-ended work may yet get a chance, someday.

Waldron, Gazzilo, Stukenberg, and Gorman (2018) provide a useful summary of significant outcome research for psychoanalytic therapies that support their inclusion as treatment choices. Core conflicts are eased, but not erased, and better understanding means better coping skills. The "fit" between therapist and patient is an important curative variable, with an emphasis on adapting to the specific needs of each patient. Two findings are more supportive of analytic work than other therapies, namely the value of greater frequency and duration as well as longer-lasting effects. Frequency and duration are potential cost problems in the short term, but they do support the provision of explorative opportunities that can be linked to the relatively lasting nature of therapeutic effects. Money and effort spent now could reduce the repetitive cost of quick but frequent therapies. However, that value has at the moment insufficient appeal to potential consumers.

A result of the current exclusion of psychoanalysis is that many therapists trained as analysts cannot practice in the traditional way they were taught, creating some identity confusion. Reflecting this, Fonagy (Jurist, 2010) has noted that therapists trained as analysts will not be identified that way in their practices. However, they will retain selective psychoanalytic principles and techniques that they continue to find effective based on patients' reactions. Now analysts need to focus on the discovery and application of psychoanalytic theories and practices that prove to be successful with a variety of patients in a variety of settings as well as integrating other therapeutic approaches. For example, Waldron and coauthors (2018) did find value in both supportive and intensive approaches. Such integration usually involves revisions and expansions of the psychoanalytic field, using it as "test site" to continue to look for "what works," shaping efforts to meet diverse groups of patients. The greatest demand for services comes from clinics and hospitals where patients are not candidates for traditional psychoanalysis. There are large patient groups of severely disturbed people who have been relatively ignored by analysis. We aim to use psychoanalysis in expedient ways to treat the broad range of pathologies that exist now. This type of work is psychoanalytic psychotherapy.

Psychoanalytic Therapy

Psychoanalytic psychotherapy has often been viewed as a limited version of psychoanalysis, with an implication that it is inferior in terms of results, and that patients using it are also limited in their personality structures relative to those in psychoanalysis. Limitations do exist in terms of the extent of possible exploration and the willingness of participants in the lengthy, extensive, and expensive process of psychoanalysis. However, rather than focusing on what is not going to happen, it is helpful to utilize what can happen in a mode of psychoanalysis that can be designed for a much larger group of people. As mental health providers, our aim needs to be developing the most effective treatment for people who need it, not designing the most powerful treatment for the smallest number of people who can take advantage of it. Furthermore, such a concentration tends to restrict concepts, theories, and practices to one group that neglects to do the best for most people. In contrast, flexibility, adaptation, expansion, and integration are necessary now on a broad scale. The test for the value of psychoanalysis will be the degree to which it can be used in some fashion to improve the treatment of the increasing number of people who need help.

Currently most people in need of treatment are unwilling, unable, or uninterested in meeting the demands of "pure" psychoanalysis. To regain status as a significant treatment option for a substantial number of patients it has to be viewed as more *relevant*. This means emphasizing what it can contribute to psychotherapy rather than focusing on what can seem to be esoteric elements of psychoanalytic practice. The relevant contributions now can be its theories of personality development and formation as well as the practical understanding and application of unconscious motivations. Psychoanalysis can continue in many ways to be considered an intriguing type of psychotherapy for a relatively small number of patients, thereby reducing its general relevance, or it can be considered a large-scale theory of human development with selective applications that are considered psychoanalytic theories and therapies. These will vary in their emphasis and desired effects, determined by each patient's expressed needs and degree of satisfaction in having their needs met. These therapies are integrative, though with a psychoanalytic foundation open to other theories, ideas, and procedures, the emphasis being "what works."

Identity Diffusion/Confusion

What is being suggested is that it is most appropriate for people trained as analysts, and open to practicing with all people in need of mental health treatment, to describe themselves as "psychoanalytic psychotherapists" rather than "psychoanalysts," while still retaining their personal identity as psychoanalysts. Etezady (2018) comments, "Whether parochial and elite or eclectic and practice-minded . . . we strive toward increasing integration and a more holistic viewpoint" (p. 2). Parochial and elite are primarily associated with psychoanalysis, while eclectic and practice-minded indicate psychoanalytic psychotherapy. "Elite," meaning "special," remains a favorite for personal retention as a self-concept, given all that went into attaining that title, but being practice-minded is indeed just fine, and in fact, relevant. The practice is psychoanalytic psychotherapy, integrative but with a psychoanalytic core, and it continues to include psychoanalysis, but the opportunities for that are much less.

This is a modification in service of contemporary practice, and training will need to expand to take this into account in considerable detail in the future, but the emphasis of the moment is to be able to survive and thrive, which requires fealty to improvement rather than tradition. Designing an appropriate place within this moving structure of adaptive treatment is complicated by ambivalence to what can seem like "pop-up" pluralism just when a position has been established, but such is the price of what can seem like unfettered growth. This is a period of adjustment to the discomfort of being trained to do one thing and most often doing another, yet employing a basic connection that is a personalized version of psychoanalytic therapy. Indicative of such a shift are surveys of relatively current psychoanalytic practices (Cherry et al., 2009; Crecci, 2010) showing that although trained as psychoanalysts, most of their practices consisted of once-a-week patients.

Endorsing this reversal from analysis to therapy provides a pragmatic evolution for psychoanalysis which assuages some of its practical problems as well as conceptual errors. Training purposes can have continued valuation of duration, intensity, and depth while supporting continual conceptual reevaluation. While there is always more to be learned about the self, there is not always an inclination to do it, even if the analyst thinks it is the best course over time for a patient. Psychoanalysis remains possible for those who have the resources to use it, but its current relevance is the foundation for psychoanalytic therapy.

An example of how this can work on a clinical level is the book by Renik (2006), *Practical Psychoanalysis for Therapists and Patients*. The value of psychoanalytic concepts for treatment is demonstrated in the book by Aron and Starr (2013), *A Psychology for the People: Toward a Progressive Psychoanalysis*. Other authors have suggested integrating psychoanalysis with other therapies (Levenson, 2010; Summers & Barber, 2010; Wachtel, 1977). Recently Busch (2018) has posed a strong alteration emphasizing behavioral change.

The Personalized Approach

Although psychoanalysis has diversified to include theories of behavior, of culture, of the mind, and other possibilities, it did begin as a method to make people feel better, a treatment for mental illness. In its development it has involved entanglements regarding the degree that theory and practice inform each other, given that ideally therapists have theories underlying their practices. Although intertwined, there are distinctions between theory of practice issues, as frequency of sessions, and theories of personality structure, as separation-individuation. Psychoanalytic therapists offer treatment based on psychoanalytic concepts, primarily that unconscious developmental disturbances lead to subsequent personality disturbances that are likely to be modified through both insight and the relationship with the therapist. Such therapy does involve modifications in frequency and duration as well as a focused use of concepts such as defenses and transference. Also involved are changes in concepts that have been altered over time, such as the transformation of linear to nonlinear models of gender development and more active involvement by therapists. Theories of practice and structure continue their interconnection, but the content becomes altered with the treatment experience.

As trained psychoanalysts are faced with limited demand for "pure" psychoanalysis, but strong demand for psychotherapy, analysts are in the process of fashioning personal versions of psychoanalytic psychotherapy. For example, we have been doing this for some time and have come to realize we have plenty of company as most analysts are seeking effective directions. We have come to experience this process as a continuing project of on-the-job training as there has been little formal training as to how to do this or devising the formal ingredients. In many instances we are all going our ways, but sensing we have a common ground, the *psychoanalytic way*. Given that we are all offering psychoanalytic therapy, we would appear to have an idea of the psychoanalytic concepts that unify us, but, as we have demonstrated (Herron & Javier, 2019), it is proving difficult for analytic therapists to agree on these unifying elements that make all the therapies psychoanalytic.

Aron and Starr (2013) have suggested seven features drawn from a comparison of psychodynamics with cognitive therapies (Blagys & Hilsenroth, 2000). These are affective focus, patients' avoidance of disturbing thoughts and feelings, identifying patterns, developmental focus, interpersonal focus, therapy relationship, and fantasy. They consider these as differentiating analytic therapies from other therapies, but given the plethora of current treatments, these factors are questionable as being sufficiently distinctive. As nonanalytic therapies have borrowed generously from analytic, they all seem to appear to some degree in both types of therapies.

The primary distinctive feature is the emphasis on the unconscious (Aron & Starr, 2013; Morris et al., 2015; Shedler, 2010) as a motivational factor. Therapies that consider it necessary for patients to become aware of factors outside of their conscious awareness as motivators of their actions and use such awareness to alter their behavior are psychoanalytic, whereas those that strive for behavior change without such awareness. While Busch (2018) has noted that behavior change without insight can occur, therapies with such an approach are not that successful (Shedler, 2017).

At the same time, therapeutic approaches have not developed to the point that the field has arrived at the *psychoanalytic therapy*, nor is there definitive evidence to support the universal usage of psychoanalytic therapies rather than behavioral ones. The current situation does indicate there are successful psychoanalytic *therapies* with varying specifics but united in making the unconscious, conscious. Shedler

(2010) has suggested some other fundamentals, such as focusing on emotional conflict, ambivalence, influence of the past, transference, defenses, and the meaning of symptoms. Gediman (2011) has suggested defenses, resistance, the unconscious, the therapeutic relationship, transference, and countertransference. Except for the unconscious, these are not unique to psychoanalysis, but when appearing in other therapies are given other names. The point remains, however, that psychoanalysis is the prototype for all talk therapies.

Doing What Works

It now seems likely that a limited market for extensive analysis will remain active, attesting to the value of the examined mind for some people, but its current value lies elsewhere. The focus shifts to the *idea* of a better determination of results, as well as attempts to demonstrate these results, and to the correction of conceptual and practical errors. This book is about *what works*, clinical value, much of which can be found in psychoanalysis. It is learned experientially through therapeutic efforts with each patient, which is a lengthy process open to error, but necessary to produce better results. The theoretical framework being created has to fit each patient, not patients put into each therapist's favorite ideas, though ideas need to continue to be created and tested, which in turn has to mean some mistakes. Resistance is to be expected and respected along with establishing a therapeutic alliance. The first step needs to be finding out what the patient wants, not pushing the patient into what therapists find interesting and in turn would like to give, and that certainly opens the door to pluralism. Although symptom relief has been decried as less than sufficient in terms of what a patient could get, and that may be true, it will not be attained if a patient is not receptive. Many, if not most patients want relief from suffering, which means getting rid of one or more symptoms listed in some fashion in the diagnostic manual. Patients also want to know, or at least believe, that therapists can be of help and they want to know what is going to be involved. Given therapists' own uncertainty about how well their methods work and difficulties in explaining what indeed may be involved, what patients want, and what therapists can do, the match is difficult, yet needs to be attempted. Particularly in this matchmaking, the psychoanalytic foundation for therapy can be very helpful because it attempts to provide causal pathways to manifestations of psychopathology as well as approaches to feeling better.

The patient's task is to talk as freely as possible about himself (loose associations) regarding the presenting problem while the therapist's is to listen for those pathways (focused attention) as they work together for an exploration of possibilities and solutions. Such a procedure is likely to develop previously unexplored pathways, problems, and solutions as well as the apparent presenting problem, so both expansion of issues and new directions may appear. Therapy is a search for the causes of patients' problems and a search for ways for patients to behave differently to improve their lives, but it is directed toward symptomatic understanding and adaptive behavioral functioning rather than broad personality reconstruction. The procedures of classical analysis, described by Greenson (1968), remain useful descriptions of what happens in the therapy. These are confrontation, clarification, interpretation, and working through, and they were designed to be employed in a setting of free association. Now the field changes to a more focused, and less free-ranging situation where a patient describes his life with more specific problematic issues and the therapist plays a more active role in considering possible solutions. Confrontation and clarification are essentially melded so that the therapist sees contradictions as well as being an active participant in what they are both saying. There is a reactive exchange taking place, beginning with an awareness of what is being said by each one and what feelings are happening. A relationship is being developed in which the patient can feel supported in self-expression and the therapist can be relatively reactive.

From the start it is likely the patient will be ambivalent in providing self-revelation, despite ostensibly being willing to talk about personal issues. Patients are aware that therapy is designed to foster change, but there is always some resistance to change. The patient wants to be released from whatever bothers him, but at the same time wants to do what feels safe and familiar. This is a common problem in all psychotherapies. At times he will in essence want to change while being the same, which slows down the progression of the therapy and can be more acute in psychoanalytic therapy than in analysis where there is more time for detailed exploration. This puts added pressure on the therapist to respect both desires of the patient. This is a delicate proposition involving making progress while holding contradictions. Even patients who are very declarative about wanting a "new self" also want to retain certain aspects of the old self that the therapist may experience as impeding the creation of a "better self." Although therapists often have versions of the "best self" for a patient, success in psychotherapy usually means acceptance of limited improvement. The task is to facilitate the most effective self that is comfortable for the patient as support for positive changes that do occur. The patient is the ultimate guide and arbiter of what will be accomplished.

Symptom Relief

Most patients indicate they want symptom alleviation and removal if possible. Psychoanalysis has customarily offered something different, something more, basically significant life improvement which has definite appeal. Doing less than that has been depicted as damaging the analysis, but psychotherapy often does not provide the time and environment for extensive personality exploration. Although psychoanalysis got its start as symptomatic treatment, over time that goal seems to have been overshadowed by more ambitious aims. For example, considerable emphasis has been given to patient improvement through a better understanding of the mind. Fred Busch (2014) has emphasized the creation of a psychoanalytic mind including two types of knowledge, *state* and *process*. The former enables a patient to know what had been unknown and the latter is an understanding of the process of understanding. The patient becomes a better thinker and in turn a curative process occurs, but the emphasis appears to be on creating the psychoanalytic mind rather than the behavioral result which seems to be depicted as inevitable if indeed the process has created a psychoanalytic mind. He takes note of the "essential creative process" being the patient creating a capacity for reflection. He emphasizes the process. It is indeed detailed, extensive, and fascinating, but not practical. In contrast, Frederic Busch (2018) questions assumptions about the negative effects of disruptions in neutrality, the use of suggestion, and symptom removal, all available in psychotherapy as treatment modalities.

The shift away from treatment is more apparent in the work of Stern (2015), impressive and appealing but restrictive in application. He eschews the idea that psychotherapy (as he practices it) is a medical or scientific procedure, and he values case studies and theories as evidence of effects more than quantitative research. He does conclude that most of his patients "get better," meaning that their lives improve. However, he states "I am not willing to agree that symptomatic relief is any kind of measure of my work. I think of psychoanalytic work as the investigation, deconstruction, and creation of meaning" (Stern, 2015, p. 191).

By definition a patient is in distress, so whatever he undertakes to get relief he will consider to be treatment for the distress. For Stern's (2015) approach to have patient appeal there is a need for the probability of relief. A possibility exists as a type of footnote regarding the effects of investigation, deconstruction, and creation of meaning, but most patients want that to be a primary goal of the process, so even if the analyst has another name, or goal, for it, patients think of it as treatment. The process he is offering is lengthy and thorough, but if it is not designated as treatment that limits its relevance for patients. The elaboration of the process, with its intriguing conceptualizations, has wandered too far from the original goal of being a revolutionary therapeutic method.

The case for psychoanalysis as a treatment method requires more of an emphasis on psychoanalytic ideas regarding the development of psychopathology and its remediation procedures, such as symptomatic relief as well as personality reconstruction. Psychoanalytic methods and theories can be used in service of emotional and cognitive improvement, with the therapeutic method aimed at making a person feel better within the framework of a therapist-patient relationship that is portable to the world outside of the therapeutic setting. Such expansion is not a "byproduct" of the experience, but it is "the product" for therapist and patient.

This viewpoint may be a "hard sell" for many analysts. For example, even Wachtel (2014), an early and consistent advocate for theoretical and practical integration for psychoanalysis, comments, "As analysts what engages us most deeply are matters such as the complexity of human experience, the nuances of subjectivity, and the full human thriving, not just relief from symptoms" (pp. 51–52).

However, the patients are not therapists, so interests diverge. The complexity of human experience and nuances of subjectivity are not high on the interest list for most patients and the degree of thriving is likely to be very personalized. Relief from symptoms is what primarily engages patients and what they primarily want from most therapists, including psychoanalytic ones. The other concepts mentioned, while not defined operationally, certainly appear as useful achievements, but not obvious patient attractions.

Symptom relief may well bring changes in the way patients think and feel on a relatively broad basis, and cognitive and affective shifts are also likely to bring symptom relief, but the goals are not interchangeable. Symptoms are patients' preoccupations. For most patients now the therapeutic alliance requires more focus on symptomatic improvement than psychoanalytic therapists have been inclined to give in the past. Patients need to feel that their therapists are allied with them in understanding what the patients want. Therapists need to be viewed as having the knowledge and skill to help the patient meet the patient's goals. It appears as if psychoanalysis as a theory and practice has been drifting away from the treatment toward privileging theory. Theories are indeed of interest, but for the patient, "feeling better" is the primary goal while the examined mind is "just" a possible accompanying process.

Customized Treatment

Given the extent of mental health issues in our society, psychotherapy ideally would be an "open-access" procedure available to whoever needed it whenever they needed it and for whatever length of time it took to improve their conditions. Unfortunately, it is clear that practical issues sharply curtail such an approach. Gnaulati (2018) argues that the combination of insurance companies, pharmaceutical companies, and bad science has tarnished the appeal of classic talk psychotherapies such as psychoanalysis. By now we are all too familiar with a prevailing idea that emotional problems are best handled through brief therapies and medications despite unimpressive results. As an antidote, we put our efforts into finding ways to increase the effectiveness of psychotherapy that can be made available rather than dwell on the dismal effects of the current treatment environment. We are attempting to find ways to utilize psychoanalytic concepts and practices effectively within the field now available to us.

An example of this approach is transference-focused psychotherapy (TFP) (Yeomans et al., 2015), a manualized treatment model that describes flexible applications of transference-focused treatment adapted to patients' problems, and which has also been subject to empirical evaluation. Our efforts are less formalized but aim at being pertinent in illustrating the search for what works.

Currently patients do not have the resources for extensive treatments, so adaptation is necessary. This means reshaping whatever aspects of psychoanalysis that are required to meet the expressed needs of patients. We consider psychoanalysis to have the elasticity of psychoanalytic psychotherapy for this purpose without deviating from its basic facilitative purpose. For example, all psychotherapy involves transference, resistance, countertransference, and a therapeutic alliance, regardless of what these happenings may be called, but the degree to which these concepts will be explored will vary with each patient. This is particularly true with unconscious motivation which is the foundation for the concepts and is always involved as well. However, it is necessary to keep in mind the finding that symptoms can be reduced without patients having insight into intrapsychic conflicts and that symptom substitution is not an inevitable response (Thoma et al., 2015).

We are searching for "what works," and in so doing we encounter the need to use alterations in customary psychoanalytic approaches. In particular, we often do not have a "psychoanalytic field" to support our use of technical interventions whereas the body of work supporting the effectiveness of psychoanalytic approaches (Downing & Mills, 2017; Kernberg et al., 2008) involves patients where the treatment situation would allow more traditional psychoanalysis, but the severity of patients' pathologies requires technical variations. We do have a similar issue of treating a wide range of disturbances, but our "treatment field" is notably variable, particularly regarding the frequency of sessions, length of sessions, intervals between sessions, and patients' motivations. This means our work is significantly experimental, so we are presenting it as an invitation to comment and we view it as far from definitive, but reflective of the diffuse "fields" in which we work. We do believe that our practices reflect the existing need for psychotherapy in which psychoanalytic work can have great practical potential that rivals, or better, improves upon current situations.

Searching for "what works" is most accurately described as "what seems to work," and it usually results in modifications both in application and theory. These may be considered some type of personalized similarities, the latter being represented by the psychoanalytic link, while the latter indicates the uniqueness of the analyst's style of expression. Kernberg (2019) has suggested four basic technical applications, namely interpretation, transference analysis, technical neutrality, and countertransference utilization. Supportive techniques are an addition to these. However, Kernberg (2019) also notes that concerning the systematic use of fundamental psychoanalytic techniques the psychoanalytic field needs to permit transference development and the deepening of therapeutic information as well as interventions. In our work there are limitations on these applications, such as free association that facilitates them in the usual analytic field. Instead, the therapeutic field has to be focused on apparent patient needs and abilities. At the same time, this emphasis still tends to include unconscious motivation, consideration of different ways of thinking and feeling, intersubjectivity, influence of the past, defensive needs, relational and drive recognitions, and resistance, although the extent of exploration is limited.

As psychoanalysis has evolved it has taken a relational turn in which much has been made of the limited objectivity of the analyst, the subjective nature of interpretation, and an increased egalitarianism between analyst and patient. It has become common to describe analysis as a "co-creation" of analyst and patient. This usually implies a diminution of the analyst's power as the ultimate determiner of interpretation and a restriction of the idea that apparent insights are being analyst-inspired or created. This has been a useful pushback against the idea of an "all-knowing" analyst with extensive objectivity, but it has created some problems as well. There are two people involved, so it has always been a "co-creation," but there was a tilt that often inflated the analyst's power. The issue is creating a proper balance between patient and therapist. The patient seeks knowledge from the therapist that the patient does not have, namely a solution to some problem. The therapist is expected to supply that knowledge to the patient in some manner, so in that sense, the analyst always knows more than the patient and has been trained to have a certain detachment from the patient that permits relative objectivity. Attunement to countertransference is necessary to support the most useful subjective-objective balance.

Psychoanalytic psychotherapy involves strong guidance from the expressed needs and immediate concerns of patients. The balanced co-construction is guided accordingly with patients as the ultimate filters of importance. Therapists' input varies, with roles shifting according to patients' needs and therapist capabilities. Many patients are asking for a relatively rapid understanding of their issues, support, and pathways to solutions that mean the patients can feel better. Although there are issues and areas of each patient's personality that can be of interest to the therapist and are construed as useful for a patient to explore, only some are seen by each patient as important. Although the issue of overall mental health is important, the emphasis often has to be in favor of immediate concerns. The assistance of the therapist should be useful, but it often can only be limited, particularly regarding the extent of solutions. The underpinnings are primarily psychoanalytic, but the therapy is carried out with whatever is offered by patients. The therapy remains psychoanalytic based on the belief in the value of understanding unconscious motivation, but it utilizes a variety of theoretical and practical viewpoints. The problems of patients are viewed as being caused by a mixture of conscious and unconscious factors. Treatment involves a search for options in terms of causes and solutions, for connections between symptoms and possible causes and ways to use these connections to induce more effective patient behavior.

We often work with "neglected populations," namely patients who have been hospitalized or treated in clinics for psychiatric diagnoses, so we are particularly interested in developmental features that may have contributed to symptom patterns. Recognizing the incomplete correlation between specific developmental trauma and disorders, as well as the contribution of genetic and organic factors, and current circumstances, the probability remains that developmental experiences significantly foster subsequent behavior in a patterned manner. There are probable patterns from the past that can be clues to identifying and understanding current pathology. This view is in line with research supporting the formative importance of the developmental environment, particularly early deprivations (Mahlberg, 2018).

Although we have emphasized a psychoanalytic foundation, we consider our approach an integrative one. The ingredients are broad, but it is not being advanced as a comprehensive consensus, though we support that possibility. Also, it is more practice-driven than theory-based. It does foster explanations of behavior that have unconscious sources and the potential to lead to behavior change. The potential of theoretical causes lies in their resonating with patients, so the utility of our conception rests on patients' acceptance, although subject to possible distortions due to transference. Also, theories can be accurate, but not reach fertile ground, depending on technique, which can be appealing even if deceptive. Although these error possibilities are noted, apparent patient satisfaction remains a good source of evaluating therapeutic success. Practice-driven means using what ultimately appears to facilitate change, keeping in mind the pitfalls of evaluation. Lichtenstein (2018) stated,

"To take the subject as an object is to lose something of its character, and what is being evaluated is also a reduced and distorted version" (p. 28).

Increasing effectiveness means not only changes in technique but the retrofitting of psychoanalytic thought as well. Several psychoanalytic concepts need to be revisited and reshaped to facilitate practice in the current environment. Our coverage is likely to be incomplete, but it does provide examples where we found difficulties along with possible solutions that work for us and that we consider useful in general for the evaluation of analytic therapies and their evolution. These include pluralism, identity formation, psychic development, transference, countertransference, resistance, research, diversity, and applied psychoanalysis. We conclude with a summary of the clinical value of psychoanalysis.

Pluralism: Pathways to Integration

Pluralism is a comprehensive description of different theories and practices that exist within a particular psychology, such as psychoanalysis or CBT, as contrasted with orthodoxy that requires adherence to a specific set of theories and practices. The current state of psychotherapy has become pluralistic, both in psychoanalytic (Herron & Javier, 2019) and behavioral (Hayes et al., 2004) traditions. However, this has led primarily to diversity within the approaches and dissension as to their value rather than integration.

Despite the within-discipline disagreements, emphasis remains on the use of pluralism. Within CBT, Barlow (2008) provides detailed examples while Jurist (2018) supports pluralism in psychoanalysis. Although it appears that pluralism is here to stay, opening the possibility of integration, such an approach has not been formalized. It certainly could be, as Wachtel (1977) pointed out some time ago, and the recent work of Buechler (2019) appears as an undeclared example of integration with its focus on problems in living.

We see integration as a necessary step to improve mental health services for patients, and to restore the relevance of psychoanalysis. At the same time, we understand the concern about a loss of identity that is prominent in each school and tradition of psychotherapy. As a result, rather than immediately embracing integration and working that way, we want to illustrate the path in psychoanalysis that has brought it to the recognition of the current pluralism.

Pluralism in Psychoanalysis

Although orthodoxy was emphasized in psychoanalysis, there were always conflicting views. In 1958 Rapaport was attempting to develop a comprehensive theory of psychoanalysis, but he abandoned the effort due to the extent of existing diversity. At the same time psychoanalysis was considered to be a unified theory. It was not until the publication of *Object Relations in Psychoanalytic Theory* by Greenberg and Mitchell in 1983 that there was official room for theories other than Freud's drive theory that included modifications such as ego psychology. The recognition of object relations theory, however, did not result in integration with drive theory. Instead, there has been competition among the theories as to which was truly "psychoanalytic."

For example, Pine (1990) described an integration of four notable psychoanalytic psychologies; drive, ego, object, and self. His approach is an additive one, seeing the new approaches as building on the old as well as making corrections in existing theories and practices. While some dissenters want a "new psychoanalysis," the main current approach is accepting pluralism in an attempt to bring together the strengths of the different viewpoints around a common core. While we opt for the unconscious in that regard (Morris et al., 2015), there remains a lack of consensus as to what is the essence of psychoanalysis and a comprehensive theory of psychoanalysis continues to be elusive.

The result is the acceptance of pluralism with loose connections among its various practitioners who share the identity of being psychoanalysts. The identity is usually solidified by the practitioners having trained in psychoanalytic institutes and sharing the use of some psychoanalytic concepts, such as unconscious motivation. This sharing of diversity, and its acceptance, does increase the possibility of greater relevance for psychoanalysis. There is an openness to more potential patients, but the openness does not extend to nonpsychoanalytic therapies. Of course, the latter are not open to psychoanalysis, instead seeing themselves as distinct and more effective. At the same time, both approaches use concepts from each other without acknowledgment and use different names for the concepts. The lines of distinction are blurred, but not formally crossed in most instances.

We identify as psychoanalysts who are interested in the integration of non-psychoanalytic approaches. This is congruent with the work of Wachtel who has written extensively about its value while maintaining his analytic identity. As an integrationist he points out that he thinks differently about psychoanalytic concepts yet retains his interest in them and his attention to them. He believes in dialogues, integration, and openness to new approaches, and sees such an attitude as the path to progress in psychotherapy. So do we. The differing viewpoints that exist in pluralism offer the opportunity for listening to others, considering possible clinical values for patients, and being open to using alternative approaches. Wachtel (2011) elaborates on points of convergence, noting that CBT has moved away from a strictly rational approach where the lack of rationality is considered the source of psychopathology, that replacing the irrational with the rational is effective, and that this can be easily accomplished. Instead, CBT has become more effective and acceptance-centered. This converges with psychoanalytic concerns with affective experience and the acceptance of apparently unacceptable tendencies within the self. There is an awareness of unconscious processes and life-span developmental experiences as well as the interaction between the self and the social, interpersonal environment. There is also an awareness of the importance of the therapeutic relationship and the influence of developmental processes.

Wachtel's cyclical psychodynamic theory is designed as an integrative psychotherapy. It considers the influence of unconscious motivations, creation of conflicts, defenses, and symptoms, but is relatively oriented toward present experiences such as how emotions are regenerated in a self-perpetuating process. The starting point for disruptive emotions may be in the past, but it is maintained in the present despite conflict and ambivalence. In essence, pathology is both desired and not desired and is contextual. There are both negative and positive cyclical patterns, with the thera-peutic effects occurring through building the patients' strengths.

Anxiety is seen as a learned reaction to fear of fundamental desires, with ther-apy focusing on helping patients overcome that reaction. The primary focus is not on the content of the fear, but the reason for the anxiety and methods to overcome it. Behavior therapy suggests exposure, but psychodynamic approaches make expo-sure indirect via interpretation, leading to control and feeling safe. A basic aim is to help patients integrate their experiences so that what had previously evoked anxiety now becomes an acceptable understanding of the functioning self.

Pluralism provides options. One, relatively narrow, is to have a new and dif-ferent view within the scope of a particular therapeutic approach. An example is considering relations more important than drives, but remaining within the psycho-dynamic orbit. It took courage to adhere to such a view in the distant past but is now quite acceptable. This is a significant opening in the psychoanalytic field. Inte-grating that with more traditional concepts rather than displacing the possibilities of instinctual drives as motivations also represents pluralism and retains more of the psychoanalytic tradition. Other types of pluralism include additive and displac-ing, both currently active and likely to be acceptable within the psychoanalytic view. However, while likely to be utilized more than traditional analysis, it is unlikely that any of the pluralism depicted so far is sufficiently practical for a significant num-ber of potential consumers. As long as a therapist maintains a significant attach-ment to a particular brand of therapy, the therapist tends to adhere to the treatment approach of that therapy, regardless of what the patient wants.

This does not mean a disregard for the patient, but rather a belief that the ther-apeutic method being used is the most curative measure. If a therapist replaces one allegiance for another, the issue is the relative influence of the method. For example, describing the therapy as co-constructed means that the input of both parties will be shaped to fit the therapist's view of what is most helpful. If, in the therapist's view, the patient is not "constructing" to fit the therapist's model, it will be considered resistance. The "looser" the therapist's model, the greater the patient's influence, but, patients do not go into therapy to tell the therapist how to solve the problems that brought them there. There is always, by design, a tilt. It is expected by the patient, and it is in the direction of the therapist's expertise.

Psychoanalytic therapists are trained to attract patients to their approach, based on a belief in its value, but their approach may not be congruent with the patient, so the burden of retention falls on the therapist. The mismatch is an argument for going beyond pluralism with theoretical boundaries to being open to integration. Buechler (2019) makes the point that although therapists are trained to be neutral no one is really neutral. Neutrality is like co-construction, relative and contextual. Psychoan-alytic therapists are trained to work on character structure with the belief that will benefit patients more than immediate symptom relief, but many patients want the symptom relief first, and maybe, later, character alterations. Granted "immediate" relief is unlikely regardless of methodology, but symptom mitigation is a faster pro-cess than character alteration. Buechler (2019) illustrates the problem confronting psychoanalytic therapists who are frequently working with patients trying to solve problems in living, such as uncertainty, aging, loss, and solitude, among others. It is basic stuff, now stuff, and they want to help in finding answers.

Pluralism opens the door, not to anything goes, but to seeking answers to what hurts now. There is an avoidance of advising patients even though patients ask for it frequently. The implication is that mental health is equated with the ability to make personal decisions rather than being told what to do by someone else. However, in this case, someone else is a mental health professional, which means therapists have skills the patient does not have, but these skills do not necessarily include how a patient should lead life. They do include an awareness of productive life skills as well as methods to acquire and use such skills. Thus, direct advice, such as what the patient should do in a particular situation, could be inaccurate because the therapist is not an expert in living life. Countertransference is always a possibility. Therapists themselves struggle with life, feel anxious, get depressed, suffer loss, age, have physical illnesses, make mistakes, and essentially have many of the problems that their patients have. Therapists are not automatically good models of mental health, though they certainly should try to be. Unfortunately, personal therapy is no guarantee of this, but it can help.

Along with personal therapy, which is guaranteed with analytic therapists, psychotherapy training does provide learning about how people develop and behave. This includes what works for them and what does not, as well as methods that result in positive behaviors. These are paths to a fulfilling life as well as possible obstacles. Therapists have a heightened awareness of these concepts. Pluralism in regard to theories and practices is a useful way to learn what is available and to develop what appears to be most useful.

Consider Beuchler's (2019) response to the question of what she, as a therapist, can offer patients who want help with life challenges such as loss, aging, suffering, and shame. "I believe I can bring my life experience, my clinical experience, and use insights drawn from theory. . . . It helps me conceptualize some fundamental issues . . . reformulate the questions . . . reformulating dilemmas is the clinician's contribution to the patient's struggle toward personally resonant responses to life's predicaments" (p. 4).

Integration

Integration is the ultimate pluralism where steps are taken to differ from the customary parameters of the therapist's declared orientation. Wachtel's theory of cyclical psychodynamics is a significant example of pluralism as integration. By maintaining his basic identity as a psychoanalyst but using other approaches as well, his emphasis is on what works. Therapy is designed to fit each patient rather than each patient fit the rules of a designated theory. Psychotherapy becomes very much patient-centered as pluralism expands to integration with other theories and practices beyond the therapist's original designated orientation.

Cyclical psychodynamics stresses interactive repetitive cycles of connection between people that take into account the field of interaction, unconscious and conscious motivations, individual and social dynamics, and the influence of developmental factors. There is a focus on the mutual influences of past and present on each other and it elevates the importance of how the patient lives now. Although the origins may be in the past, it is the interactive present that keeps the patient's problems alive. However, the dynamics of repetition are not viewed as an intention to repeat, but resulting from trying to avoid the repetition, and the repetition is fostered by current patterns of interaction with others. In essence, while not eliminating the possibility of repetition due to continued attempts to correctly carry out a reproduction, the emphasis shifts to present behavior that has unintended negative consequences.

The approach is generally additive to provide another way to look at what is happening at the same time that at the same time does not negate past discoveries. Wachtel (1977) provides an expansive view of coping with anxiety, a major issue in all emotional disorders. He indicates the normality of wanting to avoid anxiety that results in disruptions in current living and the possibility of restoration of parts of the self that have unnecessarily been devoted to inhibition. A shift is suggested from a focus on what makes the patient anxious to the intensity of the feeling and how that can be reduced. Exposure is important, but making it effective is a difficult process, whether it is carried out directly in action or through interpretation. The effective result is the creation of safety and mastery so that there can be a comfortable process of self-integration rather than a continued disturbance and need to dissociate unacceptable parts of the self.

Our point in providing a taste of Wachtel's integration efforts is to indicate that this can be carried out by all psychotherapists regardless of orientation. Our focus is on doing this coming from a psychoanalytic orientation that has been cautious about making changes. Pluralism certainly exists within psychoanalysis, but it is scarcely an acceptance of integration. For example, Eagle (2018a) has shown that there is little evidence to support the Oedipus complex. It is one of many possible versions of navigating the parent-child relationship and the development of identity. However, recently (Solms, 2021a) published an admittedly interesting paper challenging the biological origins of the Oedipus complex. He begins with a disclaimer that his paper is not intended to question the existence of the Oedipus complex or its important role in mental development, and he also notes that most psychoanalysts believe it is a "universal human phenomenon" (Solms, 2021a, p. 563). We hope that is not the case.

Pluralists are becoming plentiful, but integrationists are slower to appear, which is unfortunate. The relevance of the psychoanalytic approach rests on the ability to adapt to what people need. Pluralism is a start, but it needs to go further and faster. The concepts involved have been introduced. For example, object relations were always listed as an ego function as was attachment as a form of object relations. Field theory is the synthetic-integrative ego at work. Mindfulness and mentalization are types of insight. In essence the ego functions have been singularized and turned into basic motivations such as relational theory.

Consider a basic approach in traditional psychoanalytic theory, namely conflict, anxiety, defense, symptom, and expansion. Make use of the familiar model of id, ego, and superego with id representing a set of motivations whose aim is gaining expression accompanied by satisfaction. It is not necessary to classify the degree to which motivations are conscious or unconscious, but to understand that personal awareness of motivations varies, so one is always operating from partial awareness. Thus the basic psychoanalytic idea of possible unconscious influence is acknowledged. The basics are, what do I want (id), what is available (ego), and what is acceptable (superego). The reasons for "wanting" will vary. They begin with the start of the formation of the person, so at that point they are primarily body-based, and they become more complex as the environment expands to create a psychological-behavioral field, life space. The drive-relational controversy appears ensnared in a search for a generalized, perhaps universal impetus, but it appears to us that more is plausible if the desire is viewed as singular yet shared, essentially specific due to its variations, at times widespread, even appearing universal, but with varying priorities. For example, one could ask if people feel hunger universally. The answer would be, probably most people frequently, but not all the time, or to the same degree. All the "needs" have limits, exceptions, usual and unusual patterns. The search for universality, and reductionism, is a practical one, but issues such as drive versus relation, while of interest, can get in the way of individualized understanding. That is messy, but the crux of successful psychotherapy.

Given the variability of desires, influenced by bodily and environmental possibilities, let us look at what the ego has to offer. According to Auchincloss and Samberg (2012) ego functions include "cognition, perception memory, motility, affect, language, symbolization, reality testing, evaluation, judgement, impulse control, affect tolerance, representation, object relations, and defense" (p. 69).

This is a menu for operationalizing desire, though there is no mention of drive as it is the domain of the id, but object relations are on the list, although now that also could be considered a drive, and attachment is part of object relations. Attachment is part of object relations. Mentalization is part of cognition, and a case could be made for recognition as well. In essence, most motivational theories rely on ego functions and ego strength or ego weakness are important. The therapeutic issue becomes how people develop and use what reality has available. In turn, it is necessary to include the entire field of the patient, the reality of the patient and of the therapist, and the degree of congruence.

Influencing both patient and therapist perceptions of reality, and getting incorporated into the perceptions, are the superego functions of cultural, social, and moral values. These can vary over time and among individuals and are both conscious and unconscious. The superego functions are primarily experienced as "shoulds," existing as partners with what a person wants to do as well as what a person can do.

In terms of building on the existing base of psychoanalysis, it is useful to disengage from exclusivity concerning id, ego, and superego functions. There is considerable overlap because the ego has an executive function of integrative action. It is also useful to consider the focus of personality components along with the overlapping structures. Personality structure can be understood as id, ego, and superego working together to form a whole person and the self-structure can be viewed as composed of the interaction of desire, awareness, and direction. While pluralism provides the opportunity for conceptual clarity as well as new concepts, much of the derivative material is already there. We realize that what we have described is a metapsychology, and that idea is unacceptable to some theorists, as are the components we have mentioned. However, psychoanalytic approaches are theoretical plans with concomitant techniques. We are not postulating what we described as *the* way to operate. We are indicating psychoanalytic thought and method already have a lot to offer, so use them in whatever way works to help patients.

Returning to anxiety, defense, and symptoms, the sequence appears appropriate though the level of awareness seems more transparent than suggested in the past. Behavior becomes an issue when it results in feelings that are in conflict. Issues such as whether the conflict is between structures, such as ego and id, can be used, but do not have to be. The idea of a metapsychology can be useful but is not essential to conflict resolution. Patients usually arrive for treatment at a symptomatic level, so they experience conflict and attempts at defense, with defensive failure resulting in symptoms. Their level of awareness of the origins and defenses varies as unconscious components play their part in symptom formation but may well be more available to consciousness than traditionally formulated. The repetition compulsion often is apparent and can be understood as attempts at symptom alleviation.

It seems that psychoanalytic theory already provides the concepts necessary to understand psychopathology and to provide treatment. However, these concepts need refinement and elaboration. The information provided by Eagle (2018a, 2018b) is a major help in understanding specific viability. Retrofitting needs to be based on evidence as to what works, and patient progress is the ultimate evidence. The various psychologies that have appeared are attempts at underpinning successful treatment, but lean in the direction of what can be considered the "Freud error," namely exclusivity, although there is no definite comprehensive psychoanalytic system. Pluralism shows that such a system is not possible at this time, but retrofitting is continuous. As a result, we consider some recent attempts that illustrate how existing psychoanalytic theories can serve as a base for current improvements.

Drive Reconsidered

Drive theory has frequently been considered a basic motivational concept in classical psychoanalysis. It is frequently contrasted with relational theory in contemporary psychoanalysis. As the relational approach gained traction the concept of drive energy and an economic point of view has faded. However, Solms (2021b) takes the view that drive theory is a viable foundation for psychoanalysis provided that it is revised. The basic revisions he suggests are that drives are conscious, drive energy is quantifiable, there are more than two drives, and all drives are self-preservative. He concludes that there is no death drive and that Freud was incorrect when he equated sexual maturity with genitality, given the presence of alternative mature sexual lifestyles. In addition, he asserts that pleasure is not the goal of a drive but is the predictor of satiation which is the goal of the drive. Satiation is considered the ideal state as evidence of drive satisfaction. The repetition compulsion was an attempt to reduce uncertainty and adhere to the reality principle and is, in turn, an ego weakness. Freud correctly thought of mental energy as quantity but thought it could not be measured. Solms and Friston (2018) indicate it can be measured, which could provide a unifying principle for somatic and mental events. This offers the possibility of a more accurate predictive model of how the mind functions.

The drive model suggested by Solms is offered as one illustration of existing psychoanalytic theory that can be developed from its origins. In the revised version the author also offers support for an awareness of the limitations of the psychosexual stages and the development of gender identity. These concerns are a part of our approach so the main takeaway for us is the possible use of the concept of psychic energy and its employment in clinical situations. Behavior can be considered as a function of desire and energy, and desire likely requires fuel to be both activated and function over time. Consider the possibility that both the mind and body use energy that is discharged in their activities and requires replenishment for ongoing and future behavior. The duration of activity for each person varies in the methods and terms of replacement and activation. It exists for the life span but is subject to the variability of bodily functions involving a reformulation of psychic energy as a clinical application that has been suggested by Solms (2018).

In any action then we could consider the desire to carry out behavior as well as the availability of the energy to do it because the interaction effects the degree of success. Also involved is the reality of the situation, namely the availability of the ingredients of the desired action, as well as fantasy if reality is not amenable. Psychic change depends not only on learning to act and feel and act in a way that works but also on the interaction of wish and available energy to feel and act that way. The id-ego-superego conception is the underlying presence along with the fuel of psychic energy. The result of such theorizing is to support our impression that the psychoanalytic foundation is there for effective modification.

Another Step Away

Shulman (2021) offers a provocative overview of the utility of Freud's theories that suggest a number of them are inaccurate. He illustrates the inaccuracies primarily through Freud's emphasis on the importance of the psychosexual stages. Our interest is in using a model to reliably understand developmental progress, and the psychosexual stages represent a long-standing example of such a model. It is one of the past-present links that might explain symptomatic behavior. It offers etiological possibilities that, if accurate, could be very helpful in treatment. There are undoubtedly other ways to attempt this, the psychosocial stages involving separation-individuation being another example. Attachment theory is a variation of the stage approach, using types of attachment rather than stages. This approach has considerable potential for providing etiological information but needs consistent reformulation or it is a trap for predetermined restrictive interpretations. At the same time, it is an existing guideline for evaluative revisions.

Shulman (2021) explores the boundaries of durability by offering ideas of Freud that have retained visibility. This is a significant step toward accuracy, but what he then considers "elemental ideas," seem to have similar problems to those he doubted. For example, personally meaningful themes to determine dream content are plausible explanations, but this is just one way to consider dream content. It is interesting, intriguing, but very subjective. Dreams probably tell personal stories, and interpretations agreed upon by an analyst and patient may be accurate, but other interpretations exist. The same is true for unconscious intentions. The belief expressed by Shulman (2021) that "everything a patient says, does, and experiences is meaningful and intentional" (p. 1108) also requires qualification.

The magnitude and power of the unconscious appear to have more limitations than originally described. The vulnerability of childhood could well be matched by old age. In essence Freud had many good suggestions, but offered limited supporting evidence, and as well documented by Eagle, psychoanalysis has some way to go to present itself as a relevant treatment procedure. This issue is of particular relevance to our emphasis on the need for developing what works. Both the examples cited pertain to traditional analysis, but retrofitting is just as necessary in contemporary analysis. Also, the need for research evidence is only part of the story. Proof of theories ultimately rests with successful clinical practices.

Solms (2021a) states "the *clinical situation* remains best suited for determining and refining the utility of new psychoanalytic theories" (p. 1081). Shulman (2021), referring to psychoanalysis, concludes "If it (psychoanalysis) is to endure as a clinical practice, its practitioners must continue to unite its ideas with their daily application in our work with patients" (p. 1109).

Although the modifications we have just described do illustrate retrofitting, their application appears more designed for traditional analysis than the type of therapy more commonly needed. In essence, they are a move in a direction, but a bigger question remains. How can theoretical shifts get utilized in the current practical psychotherapy world? To make psychoanalytic approaches sufficiently relevant they have to apply to what we will call "symptomatic demand."

The issue of relevance goes well beyond the traditional approach. Consider the concept of intersubjectivity, articulated by Benjamin (2018) as a capacity for understanding the subjectivity of another, and the idea of a *third*, eventually a state of mutuality where there is an ongoing state of recognition. How does a therapist use those theoretical conceptions when a patient asks a basic question such as, "How do I get less anxious?" An intersubjective approach to humanity, each person a subject and an object aiming for mutual understanding is appealing as a vital endeavor of humanity, but it needs practical support. The more patient-friendly interpersonal approaches enhance flexibility, though whatever the psychoanalytic approach it should be practical if it is going to gain relevance. Relevance means the patient attends to it, makes use of it, feels something, notices, and mentalizes. Our task is to have a psychoanalytic approach that does something for most mentally ill patients. Indeed, can this be?

It has to be, not every utterance or pause, but enough. To do this in our opinion means an openness to being integrative, which means a greater openness to behavioral approaches combined with a basic analytic framework. Given the pluralism now existing in psychoanalysis without consensus for a comprehensive theory, retrofitting has stayed primarily within a psychoanalytic model. This limits

its applicability and relevance. The model needs to be integrative, embracing the entire field of inquiry and attuned to the presenting needs of patients, particularly symptom alleviation. Symptoms are both powerful cues to etiology and obstacles to attempting self-scrutiny. For example, it is difficult to get beyond a search for relief to consider causality, so "analysis" pales compared to distraction or a pill, even if those solutions are tenuous or momentary, which is frequently the case. If we want patients to pay attention to their inner selves, we have to find ways to get their outer selves to listen and focus.

Distinctions from Traditional Psychoanalysis

Our approach differs from traditional psychoanalysis both conceptually and operationally. The idea of integration is a significant difference in both areas. Conceptually we begin with motivation. The idea of relative exclusivity, namely one or two major motivations, as drive or relational theory, limits the understanding of the complexity of each person. Lichtenberg (1989) and Pine (1990), both already mentioned, appear to be aligned with our view of multiple motivations, though such a viewpoint has not been dominant in psychoanalysis. At this point we cannot be definitive in naming all possible specific motivations. Our impression is that people use a "safe harbor" approach to behavior. They seek what appears to be the most comfortable action on a feeling level. This is not necessarily "safe" behavior in the usual connotation of safety because it may involve acting out, danger, or some type of self-destruction, but it is judged by the person at the time to be necessary, and in turn, satisfying, for that person.

We consider the concept of psychic energy as useful and energy discharge being a universal motivation. The idea that thought and emotion involve energy appears accurate, as does the idea that energy is used up at times and requires restorations. In those terms psychic energy is physical energy and the mind and body appear to be constructed to use and restore energy in a relatively continuous cycle of availability.

Regarding psychic development, we believe there are developmental stages, but with more diversity and overlap than has been indicated in the psychosexual stages. Early development is certainly important, but subsequent stages can also be quite significant. Trauma in one stage can be overcome, but trauma in another stage can be quite significant. Also, some patients seem to "hang on" to early trauma, such as parental neglect, and continue to blame it for disturbing feelings at later stages in their lives, while others seem less affected although the trauma appears similar. Also, stage tasks, such as parenthood, bring their own trauma. This has been particularly apparent to us with older patients who are not at all prepared for aging and the demands of the ironically termed "golden years."

As a result, the norm appears to be numerous possibilities for emotional difficulties over time, many influenced by earlier trauma, but not necessarily to the extent that has often been hypothesized. The probability lies in the buildup of both strength and weakness over time matched with the intensity of the current event's general emotional impact. Also, where there are repetitive disturbances the concept of regression often appears, but the regression does not have to be to infantile stages. Defenses are developed when a person experiences the need for psychic protection and are retained as long as they are experienced as helpful.

The concept of identity, particularly gender identity, was linked to the development of the Oedipus complex. However, as convoluted as that could get, particularly for females, the development of identity is very complicated. If anything, Oedipus was simplistic, and inaccurate, particularly as a generalization. Biology offers the initial identity, which has been quickly reinforced by the culture, but subsequent identification is very dependent on the environment. Biology is destiny only to the extent that it has certain gender-specific functions and limitations. As a result, there is a mixture of influences, with biology accompanied by environmental influences dominating, but at times the social factors move people to alter the physical characteristics and the usual roles that would accompany the original physical designations. Also, identifying as a man or woman is partially a function of sexual desire and fantasy which has a biological connection as well as a social one. In addition, sexual desire can be experienced and acted upon with social conformity to biological sexual roles. The original idea of polymorphous-perverse sexuality, deleting the "perverse" appears to be accurate, with specifics resulting from subsequent environmental factors, primarily major objects of identification and the social environment.

Diagnosis

We are concerned with the patient's current condition, so that means establishing a diagnosis, hypothesizing as to etiological factors, and developing a treatment plan. Given that most patients are using insurance coverage, and often have Medicare as their primary coverage, this means we are using ICD-10 for the diagnostic codes. This is descriptive, symptom-based, and as Yalch (2020) points out, does not consider the possible psychodynamics of the disorder. As a result, we use our experience and awareness of the possibilities to establish a psychodynamic formulation. Detailed conceptualizations are available; for example, *Psychodynamic Diagnostic Manual*, second edition (Lingardi & McWilliams, 2017), and useful if time is available. If not, which is usually our situation, we utilize what we know of the possible dynamics involved in different symptom patterns. Most symptom patterns do involve anxiety and/or depression, for example, even a psychotic symptom such as hearing voices can be viewed as the personal creation of a person who has intense anxiety about dealing with the real world so in turn creates a world of its own. That world is often harsh and critical and reflects still another level of affect suggesting a need for punishment. If that world is pleasant, then it reflects different desires. It is a defensive position and provides possible interpretive understanding. The interpretations suggested here are only some possibilities. Another example is that obsessive-compulsive symptoms are often used to control unacceptable affects, particularly aggression. These examples are not "for sure" correlates, but they are strong possibilities, so useful as explanatory hypotheses to explore.

On a broader level, specific attachment styles developed as a function of actual experiences can result in disorganized attachment. The subsequent result can be problems in social adjustment and pathogenic beliefs (Gazzilo et al., 2020). This conceptualization can lead to therapeutic approaches that link attachment theory (analytic) with Control Mastery Theory (Gazzilo et al., 2020). We are inclined to combine psychic exploration with symptom-reduction techniques.

In line with this there is an interesting naturalistic study, with limitations such as the sample being only Italian analysts, which indicates their patients were not classical analytic patients, but rather were characterized by borderline-level defenses. Also, there was an emphasis on the present therapeutic relationship and on affective exploration that did not fit the psychoanalytic prototype (Colli et al., 2020). There was a total sample of 101 analysts, divided into three groups based on the therapists' intentions, and the results tended to support heterogeneity in line with a recent trend reported by Ablon and Jones (2005) that psychoanalysts in current practice also use techniques of nonpsychoanalytic therapies. Such integration appears to be an overlap of theoretical orientations that could lead to technical changes. Colli et al. (2020) note that one cluster of psychoanalysts conceptualized patients' pathogenic beliefs as a target, which appears to be a behavioral approach and in line with integrative therapy.

The result of the appearance of integrative approaches where analysts are doing the integrating suggests that some of the usual psychoanalytic procedures may no longer be appropriate. A useful way to illustrate the possible variations is to compare what we are proposing with the traditional practices and alterations described by Summers and Barber (2010) in their pragmatic psychodynamic psychotherapy model (PPP). PPP reflects an awareness of the need for integration but is not as extensive as the work of Wachtel, nor does it attempt to sort out the effectiveness of traditional psychoanalytic conceptions, as the limitations of psychosexual stages. However, in summarizing the development of psychotherapy over time, they note the increased customizing of therapies and the direct treatment of symptoms.

Free association, the basic technique of traditional psychoanalysis, is the first issue to be addressed. The "free" part is particularly apt in all talk therapies because it highlights the value of accurate and inclusive disclosure on the patients' part to enable therapists to understand patients' problems. However, when it is coupled with "association" it becomes a more complex task and is often met with resistance. The line from free-associating to discussing presenting problems, no less solving them, is far from being obvious to many patients. As a result, PPP uses open-minded techniques that do not have a specific aim but are present-focused. We often take it a step further because we most often find patients focused on what is bothering them. In particular, patients want to know about ways to alleviate their symptoms (this includes patients who gain from being symptomatic). By being open to what the patients state they want we encourage detailed description, which in turn results in discussing current thoughts and feelings, as well as those in the past. The process continues in the direction of the background of their feelings and thoughts, events where feelings in particular have previously appeared. We are embarking on a search for possible etiologies, and in turn, taking considerable mystery out of the psychopathology. Patients appreciate the contextual nature of this, the explanatory possibilities for symptoms. They become more open to the idea of certain thoughts and feelings having a significant impact on their behavior.

Developmental explanations are hypotheses and can be met with resistance, particularly if understood by patients previously in a different manner, so change could be required to solve their difficulties. Repetition compulsion is likely based on connections to familiar understanding and behavior, even if it has been ineffective, so the resistance can enable the persistence of symptoms. We explain to patients that staying with what feels safe although at the same time disturbing is understandable, but will not change what bothers them. We offer the idea of new behaviors, indicating improvement is phasic, takes time, appears, can again disappear, but also return and stabilize. We are supportive, encouraging, and respectful of their struggles.

We explain that personality is layered with experiences and that new experiences do not erase the old. This has been well described by Weinberger and Stoycheva (2020) in their extensive work on the unconscious. Our message to patients is that what can be expected as we work together are usually temporary periods of symptomatic relief to be extended over time until the patient feels good enough for enough time to consider themselves improved. Our method is essentially *targeted associations* designed to heighten awareness of the need to use whatever means patients find effective in this regard, including behavioral measures such as thought blocking, or anxiety medication. We also indicate that such solutions are likely to be temporary and make sure patients recognize that, so they are aware that more work needs to occur. Our overall impression is that emotional insight and a therapeutic alliance are the necessary substantive ingredients for the best results. At the same time, resistance is always a factor, so the patience of both therapist and patient is important. Where symptomatic improvement comes slowly, if the patient accepts the possibility of symptomatic reappearance, an acceptable level of improvement can be attained and maintained. We are clear with patients that symptom reduction, rather than symptom removal, is the most likely outcome.

Although symptom alleviation is the most obvious goal, it is the path to that goal which in turn involves considerable personal exploration and understanding by the patient. The result is personality alterations where attributes such as intersubjectivity and mindfulness become apparent. There are varying degrees of personality reconstruction taking place. One patient described the process as, "So this is what a new life looks like." This is the psychoanalytic process, developmental, contextual, and reconstructive. It is also refashioned to meet current mental health challenges.

The next technique for comparison mentioned by Summers and Barber (2010) is the relationship between the therapist and the patient. A therapeutic alliance has always been considered vital for therapeutic success, but what varies from traditional analysis is the degree and type of activity by the therapist. In traditional work it is understood that is to encourage patients to free associate and allow transference to develop and be interpreted. In PPP there is more of a focus on the alliance, namely making sure that the two people are working together to accomplish what the patient is seeking. The therapist is relatively active, particularly concerning current reality and the ongoing process. Our approach has a definite relational cast to it that is in line with PPP. Suggested ingredients are consistent attunement to current feelings, open negotiating of the patient and therapist roles and transparency, and an active approach with awareness of the mood of the therapy.

Summers and Barber (2010) indicate that a major focus is on current reality, particularly relational issues, though they are aware of transference issues and process them where they are appropriate to current issues. We find that although the presenting problem is of immediate concern, it tends to be linked to the past. There is usually a transferential component to the linkage, but exploring that is not always of interest to the patient. As a result, although transference, countertransference, and resistance are always present, the degree to which they are discussed varies with what appears to be useful to help each patient handle their particular concerns.

Overall Approach

Patients have problems that exist in various forms during their life. Psychoanalysis was founded on the belief that life always involves conflicts and that people continually seek ways to resolve their conflicts. The signs of these conflicts are symptoms, such as anxiety and depression, or behaviors that are inappropriate or disturbing, such as excessive aggression. The first step in working with a patient is to have the patient tell the therapist what bothers the patient, what the patient thinks is wrong with him or her. This is a surface description, and given the presence of transference, unlikely to be a total description of the problem. It is what the patient wants to reveal at that time, but there will be more to come.

We tell the patient that therapy is a mutual process of exploring the patient's life to develop an understanding of how the patient's behavior has developed and using what we have learned, putting into practice improved ways for the patient to live. We believe the process is a lengthy one and that the success of the process is dependent on the patient's willingness to be committed to the process. Our commitment is guaranteed by our willingness to engage with the patient, but if that is insufficient for the patient, we are open to transparency. Over time a mutual understanding develops, namely the therapeutic alliance. We are trying to facilitate the patient's development of ways of thinking, feeling, and behavior that work better than what the patient does currently. We provide an encouraging, insightful partner for the patient. Our mutual goal is the patient's well-being. We are not the determiners of behavior, but we will offer possibilities for the patient to consider if needed.

We explain that the patient's behavior is essentially layered, or stacked, in that new behaviors are on top of old ones. The behavioral reservoir does not empty with every new stream. The new has an old foundation, most of which is unconscious. As a result, behavioral change is often interrupted by returning to the old behavior. The repetition compulsion is an ongoing issue, but not necessarily tied to infantile wishes. Instead, it is a return to a safe, known position that feels more attractive than attempting something else. We also make it known to patients that we believe there are motives of which the patient may be unaware that can and do influence behavior.

However, self-understanding and insight are not sufficient to change behavior. Psychoanalysis has always struggled with the "working through" phase of analysis where the insight is supposed to be translated into behavioral change. While dissatisfaction with interpretation as a therapeutic tool has led to an increase in an emphasis on the value of the relationship between therapist and patient, that relationship is not "curative" either. The possibility arises that integration with other approaches could be more effective. Examples include the modification of thoughts, beliefs, cognitions, and the development of problem-solving skills. Add to this that medication can be helpful in symptom reduction and this can allow the person to feel more comfortable attempting new behavior. Mindfulness and mentalization, which can be understood as elaborations of insight, have already become part of the psychoanalytic approach.

We explain to our patients that we are trying to help them attain a "good-enough" position in their thinking, feeling, and behavior that indicates satisfaction with their lives and that we are available to assist in supporting that for as long as they find the process helpful. Freud's (1937) paper, "Analysis Terminable and Interminable," remains an apt description of the value and duration of therapy. Practical concerns usually will determine the length and impact of the therapy, along with the motivation and skill of the participants. Although it would be very satisfactory to offer a "cure," mental health treatment is unfortunately not at that level. As a result, we offer improvement in terms of what works for each person.

The Relational Turn

In a further illustration of our approach, we consider the role of the most prominent alteration in psychoanalysis, the shift from drive as the primary motivation to relationships. The need to relate, to make contact, is considered the main focus, with drives viewed as modes of contact. In our example we are using relational psychoanalysis as depicted by Barsness (2021). He uses a quote from Aron (2012, p. 1222) which indicates that the technique is aimed at creating a relationship between therapist and patient that results in "transitional, symbolic space of thirdness and intersubjectivity." It does seem that description would be difficult for patients to comprehend as a solution to what bothers them. The basic idea is that the patient-therapist relationship will be such that it facilitates the alteration of the patient's maladaptive behavior. Barsness (2021) recognizes the "muddling" of analytic technique that has evolved with the relational emphasis and attempts clarification. Affect is important and the relationship between therapist and patient is the major change agent. This is in contrast to the traditional model of insight through the interpretation of defenses. At the same time, it does require recognition of the emotional impact of an affirming, understanding relationship. This serves as a foundation for learning to change problematic relationships.

Seven categories are noted as serving to accomplish the change; one and two are therapists' intent and stance; three, four, and five, being the manner of reflection, namely deep listening, attending to the present, patterning and linking; six and seven, being engagement, as working through and courageous speech and disciplined spontaneity.

Intent requires establishing a clear understanding of the purpose of the therapy. It appears to be enjoying the range of emotions, self-reflection and soothing, toleration of uncertainty, open thinking about the past and freedom from repetition compulsion. Exploration of the past is part of this and patients tend to be selective about this, so the therapist has to tread carefully. The therapeutic attitude is meant to be collaborative, a co-construction, but the degree of contribution from each party has to vary. The degree of collaboration is likely to be more limited by the patient so the degree of interpretive togetherness is also limited. The focus is on the need for both parties to be open to varying viewpoints. It is the patient's psyche that is being explored, though the therapist's is also being stimulated and at the same time the therapist is there to be attuned to blind spots in both the patient and the therapist. The relational approach emphasizes the mitigation of the authoritarian style of traditional analysis, but the patient is there primarily because the therapist is seen as more knowledgeable than the patient. Thus, a question is raised in co-construction as to the amount, manner, and value of the patient and the therapist contributions, a question that is not answered by the term, "co-construction," without a more detailed description. It is important to recognize the therapist's realistic authority, meaning that there should be many instances where the therapist does know more than the patient, which limits the seemingly desired co-construction desired in relational analysis. Getting the proper balance seems to be a difficult issue to resolve. It does seem to us that the therapist, as analyst, should be more knowledgeable than the patient without necessarily being condescending because the patient is there to get something more than a supportive friend. The patient is not there to learn about the analyst, or to help the analyst learn, though these may be by-products. The patient is there to get better. The analyst is there to help the patient. Co-construction needs to be applied within those boundaries.

Co-construction may have pushed the needle a bit excessively regarding countertransference of therapist superiority. There is no denigration of patients that has to be implied in the therapist-patient relationship. The atmosphere of traditional analysis may well have contained such an impression and relational analysis has mitigated it, but at times it appears as if equality of knowing is the objective of the analysis rather than making the patient better. Of course, it is important that countertransference be continually examined, and the examination of what is happening to the analyst continues with deep listening, use of the associative process and the input of the patient with the apparent transmission of the patient's world. There is certainly value in affective attunement, but it borders on a preoccupation with countertransference if the therapist believes in personal awareness of the patient's unconscious via resonance with the unconscious of the therapist. There is no empirical evidence to support this.

Relational therapists are interested in attachment, development, defenses, repetition, transference, and especially, countertransference. There is a tendency to postulate projective identification and unconscious transmission from patient to analyst, but there is no empirical support for these possibilities. The "here and now" approach can cause some patients to feel the therapy is more about the therapist than the patient, so a more balanced approach between the traditional therapeutic manner and the present emphasis seems prudent. Patterning and linking appear useful but do not have to focus on the patient-therapist relationship.

Then there is working through an analytic concept that has never been well-defined. It refers to the patient being able to translate insight gained through the analytic process into action and requires repetition to ensure learning takes place. The validity of the process rests on behavioral change. For traditional analysis the insight would have come about through interpretation. In relational analysis the patient-therapist relationship would be considered the primary agent of change. Neither approach has been particularly successful in demonstrating the process or providing empirical evidence of the value of the process, no less what "working through" constitutes in practical terms. At the same time, there is sufficient case-based evidence of behavioral change using both approaches, so we use elements of both as well as whatever other approaches seem to promote change. Relational analysts also support relatively open speech and emotional expression and are open to expressing possible mistakes. We agree with reasoned self-expression that appears helpful to the patient's therapeutic progress, and to extending the analytic model to include the importance of relationships and intersubjectivity.

What appears to be missing in both the traditional and contemporary analytic models is an appropriate recognition that insight and emotional congruence depend on altered thinking that will result in altered behavior. In both instances there appears to be an assumption that if one gains insight, namely "knows better," one will act accordingly, but that is often untrue. People act as they feel and think at given moments of time. Regrets, illustrated by negative reactions, come later. The repetition compulsion takes precedence. Thus, the goal of therapy has to be behavioral change: Think different, feel different, and act different.

Behavioral change without the underpinnings of insight and relational shifts is also insufficient. There is no compelling evidence that one type of therapy is better than another or that medication is the better solution. Existing evidence indicates that existing therapies work some of the time. Our solution is integration, using whatever works in given situations. Unfortunately, the psychoanalytic approaches are being neglected currently, and along with an emphasis on cost considerations, therapeutic possibilities are being curtailed and mental health treatment remains relatively ineffective. This book is focused on bringing the psychoanalytic component back into the picture and providing an open-ended, integrative treatment based on actual need in contrast to the "hurry-up" approach now prevalent.

Next Step

Thus far descriptions of our work have been in general, theoretical terms. Now we are going to move to the content of actual sessions. Recognizing that we have enough in common regarding our faith in psychotherapy to present a relatively unified approach, we also recognize our different styles and therapeutic settings. As a result, we are individualizing the actual dialogues between patient and therapist.

4

Session Notes and Comments

This chapter describes therapist-patient exchanges that illustrate an integrative psychotherapeutic approach. Details are altered to protect the identity of the patients. The therapist is male. Comments regarding the session are also included. These patients are not typical analytic patients, but they are the type of patients that are exerting the most demand on our mental health system. They are usually offered CBT and medication only, but we used an integrative approach based on our belief in the value of integrating the psychoanalytic view as well.

In a front-page article in the *New York Times* on August 2, 2022, there is significant criticism of polypharmacy, particularly among teenagers. This article is accompanied by suggesting the need and value of talk therapy. This welcomes public support for integrative therapy and is in accord with a major thrust of this book. However, while praising intensive therapy, the example given is dialectic behavior therapy (DBT). There is no mention of psychoanalytic therapy, although we suspect even its detractors would consider it "intensive." Instead, two studies are mentioned to support the idea that this approach is indeed the most effective available treatment. So, for analytic treatment to be relevant again, it needs to prove itself, and not with just "psychoanalytic" patients.

Case 1: Slow Motion

This patient has a presenting complaint of depression about his apparent loss of cognitive and physical abilities, such as memory and activity level. He is elderly and has been diagnosed with a serious neurological disorder. He is dubious about the diagnosis, as is his family, particularly his wife who sees his actions as volitional. He does have a history of inefficiency and limited functioning, but has always been employed and has been an appropriate provider for the family.

P: I forgot my keys yesterday.

T: How does that make you feel?

P: I suppose I am careless, that I have to pay more attention to things. (The patient avoids describing his feelings, but his tone sounds as if he accepts her comment about paying attention.)

T: Do you agree?

P: I suppose I am careless. My wife wants you to give me ways to how I can improve.

T: Ways to improve? You mean, like make a list? I suppose I could do that, but you may have thought about that yourself. Do you think that memory problems could be part of your neurological disorder?

P: I suppose, if I really have the disorder.

T: You are not sure? I believe you indicated the neurologist indicated it as a strong possibility.

P: I suppose. I don't think I have the disorder. You know, I have always been forgetful. My wife tells me I just don't pay attention to things, that I need to learn to do that.

T: A learning issue?

P: Yes, I suppose. I mean, I am a slow learner, have always been. I am a mover.

T: Yes, I see you are a careful walker. Do you ever feel you might fall?

P: Yes, I might.

T: Have you fallen?

P: Sometimes, not often, but a slip a few days ago. My wife tells me I should walk more, but I am tired. (The patient then shuts his eyes.)

T: (The patient remains silent with his eyes closed for a few minutes.) Are you tired now? (The therapist is feeling the patient wants to shut him out and that he is an unwelcome interrogator. He feels it is important to discover the source of the patient's behavior, such as possible developmental patterns and/or an immediate source, the neurological disorder.)

P: (His eyes remain closed but he responds.) No, anxious.

T: You are feeling anxious right now?

P: Yes.

T: What are you anxious about?

P: I don't know. (He opens his eyes, shifts his position, closes his eyes again, and seems very uncomfortable.)

T: Let's do something about that anxiety. (Therapist has him do deep breathing exercises. After a few minutes his eyes open and remain open. He appears more relaxed.)

P: I feel better.

T: Good. I know it is difficult to discuss what seems to be happening to you, feeling like you are slipping, or even getting worse. (The therapist has been informed by the neurologist that the disorder is progressive, but the timeline is uncertain.)

P: Let's talk about something else.

T: All right. What do you have in mind?

P: Baseball.

T: Sure. (The rest of the session is spent discussing major league baseball.)

Many issues appear in this segment. Although the patient has been referred ostensibly because he is depressed, he does not mention feeling depressed but does make it clear that he is anxious. The therapist alludes to the possible depression as "difficult to discuss," but the patient does not pick up on that, instead showing anxiety, which he also does not appear to want to talk about. The therapist shows an interest in the development of symptoms and directly aids in symptom relief. A therapeutic alliance is supported by a mutual acceptance of what can be accomplished in this session. The patient, and apparently his wife, prefer his cognitive and motility symptoms to be attributed to his customary mode of operating, mistake-prone, slow of speech and manner, both viewed as relatively acceptable problems that he should be able to overcome. His wife appears as an authoritative figure, suggesting a fondness on his part for a dominating but caring maternal figure who may give him periodic hints to increase his engagement with life, and particularly with her. The therapist has a burden well beyond "behavioral hints" in that he needs to aid the patient to acknowledge his true health status and to mitigate the probable depression, and anxiety, as the patient's functioning continues to decrease. Also, the patient will have to struggle with his wife's curative beliefs if they persist once he comes to acknowledge the true nature of his disorder. Given the degree of anxiety present, tolerance of it, and open eyes, will have to come into play more often.

A counter-transferential issue here is the potential feeling of being overwhelmed by the therapist. Part of him identifies with not being in the same situation as the patient, but another part knows it could happen to him as well. Also, if the patient's wife maintains a dominance that interferes with the patient allowing himself degrees of acceptance, such as fatigue, the therapist may find himself at odds with the patient's efforts to "cure" himself which are primarily his wife's approach. The therapist believes he should let the husband-wife dynamics play out, but is already disposed to experience her as adversarial because she appears critical of the therapist's approach.

Case 2: If Only

This patient in previous sessions has been reviewing his life in reaction to current feelings of depression and loneliness. He is trying to explain himself to himself, though not necessarily altering his current way of living, but perhaps considering some malfunctions.

P: I am wondering about this, that I have grown older and it seems as if everyone else, my siblings, for example, have moved forward but I am stuck.

T: Wondering, regretting perhaps?

P: Well, yes, perhaps, in a way, sort of.

T: What way?

P: Well, I never got married and it was because I could not have anybody I had to answer to. You know how much I value my independence.

T: You are living an independent life, and your situation seems to be a good one, secure, so no one is telling you how you have to be.

P: Yes, but this is not how I was supposed to be.

T: Oh, you were supposed to get married?

P: Yes, I mean look at my brothers, all married, have families.

T: So you regret not having created a family, not having a partner?

P: Yes, but I could not do it. (Patient gives a number of examples where he was very involved with a woman and the woman would request a gesture from him, a phone call, or spending time with her. He would suddenly feel obligated, trapped, and a loss of self, and he would end the relationship. Many of his friends were gay and he had some gay relationships himself but did not consider himself gay. These relationships did not work out, the men involved did the rejecting.) You know how I am and I have to be me and I can't be responsible for another person. (This remark is in contrast with his tendency to be generous and help others. This inclination was very much in evidence of his gay relationships in which the men involved often took advantage of him without any negative reaction on his part.)

T: We have discussed this issue in the past. You felt that you could not find a partner who would accept your independence.

P: Well, I know you talked about the idea that I could discuss my feelings with the other person and that a person could understand and accommodate my feelings, but I don't believe that could happen.

T: I don't recall you ever tried it.

P: (Laughs.) I never did. It would not happen. I know that. (He seems adamant about that. It may be that his gay desires, about which he is ambivalent, impede his relating to men and women. He believes he is supposed to be a certain way, but the alternatives, the smothering women he envisions he has had, and the shame he seems to feel about being gay, leave him feeling stranded.)

T: Well you have made a life for yourself, and there is a lot of it that you enjoy. Your siblings and their children often rely on you, and you are very giving.

P: I try to do what I believe a decent person should do, would want to do.

The therapist stays focused on the patient's strengths. A more interpretive approach could be used in this session, but the instances in the past when that has been used have consistently been resisted by the patient. He was raised by rigid parents and spent much of his life striving for norms that eluded him, while trapped in what seemed like an impossible dream, to be himself. He is proud of his independence, but lonely at times and aware of the difference between his life and the family he envisioned. His sexuality seems composed of covert, disturbing desires. Actualizing a different lifestyle appears to frighten him to the point he has trouble even conceptualizing it, no less doing it. He has a rebellion going. His stated aim, to have no one control him (which would include the therapist if he got that sense) can appear to be successful, but he is actually controlled by a part of himself that restricts his connection both to others and to varying views of himself and how he could lead his life.

What is the therapist doing for him by operating at this level? The patient has connected, and remains connected to the therapist as a significant, nonthreatening object who raises alternative possibilities, but accepts the patient's struggles and his style. The therapist likes him, as is, and that keeps the patient afloat. The therapist does struggle with an interest in interpreting the possible psychodynamics more forcibly, particularly the patient's identity and an acute awareness of the patient's tendency to cut off relations when feeling threatened.

Case 3: The Other Reality

This patient has a history of psychosis, is diagnosed as psychotic, has been hospitalized, yet has considerable insight, but enormous anxiety about dealing with reality. Her emotional condition is accepted by her family who have given sufficient financial support that she does not have to work, or even interact with the world outside of her living space. This protects her, but limits her motivation to "normalize."

P: Do you have any idea what it is like to be in a psychiatric hospital?

T: I have some idea.

P: I mean, for me. What it was like for me?

T: What was it like?

P: You know I did not want to go. They just took me. (Patient begins to cry.) I called the psychiatrist to tell her I was upset. She called them.

T: I see. She must have felt you needed to be in the hospital. What do you think?

P: I didn't. I don't. (Still crying.)

T: I see. Can you tell me what was upsetting you?

P: I had been delusional, and I stopped. (Speaking clearly now.)

T: All right. You felt bad when the delusions left.

P: Yes. I felt lost. How would I survive?

T: There are ways, but tell me about the delusions.

P: I had a boyfriend. I mean, he existed, but he was not really my boyfriend.

T: Why did you think he was?

P: He was nice to me, that's all. We worked in the same place. I was wrong. I asked him if he felt that way about me and he was surprised. He said, no.

T: (Therapist smiles slightly.) Was he nice about it?

P: (Patient smiles also.) He was. I had believed it for years, but then I saw him laughing with some woman and I got doubtful. I had to ask.

T: So, you have a sense of reality?

P: Well, yes, but I don't think I like it that much.

T: You spent years hiding out. Why do you think you did that?

P: I never really had a boyfriend. I thought about it a lot, but no one really approached me, and I was not going to try, really.

T: So you gave yourself one.

P: Yes.

T: And now he's gone, and you know he was never really what you were telling yourself?

P: Yes. Reality is hard.

T: Well, what you were doing does not seem to be the best way to make a wish come true, but there are other ways, real ways, and you don't have to go to the hospital. Wishes can be fun, but so can reality.

P: I know I have to get real.

T: You took a big step when you asked him. Perhaps part of you knew the answer, felt ready for it?

P: You think so?

T: I do. I think you are saying to reality, ready or not here I come.

P: I like that idea, but I wonder if I am ready.

T: I wonder too, but let's see. We can work together to figure out why you had to imagine a relationship.

P: I never thought I could change my way of thinking, but you seem to think I can.

T: Thinking, feeling, many changes can occur.

This dialogue took place two years ago. The therapist may seem like a cheerleader and the patient seems at a relatively low developmental level, but by keeping it simple, direct, and hopeful the patient is engaged. Over time the therapy language grows in tone, capacity, and complexity because the patient gains confidence in being understood and becoming more capable. She has never been delusional again, has friends, works, and socializes, but psychosocial and psychosexual development has not expanded to the point of having a significant other. The transference is primarily positive, but at times she does get annoyed with the therapist, so the overall relationship has significant reality involved.

Case 4: More Delusions

P: Yeah, I hear voices. I mean, I am schizophrenic. That's what schizophrenics do you know.

T: What do the voices say?

P: Sometimes that I am Jesus Christ. I know that is not true. But, what if it was?

T: He had a rough life.

P: Yeah, but he was powerful.

T: You want to be powerful, but you do not feel powerful?

P: I am not powerful. I am anxious most of the time, and depressed, no job, no friends. But I know I am not going to be Jesus Christ. I know when I am delusional, but I know it afterward.

T: So, for a brief time you are powerful.

P: Yeah, but really I am not. I have other delusions, like everybody knows what I am thinking. I believe in demons, and they make this happen. They ruin my life.

T: Why you?

P: (Patient laughs.) Yeah, why me? I am nobody and who cares what I am thinking. Ridiculous, I know, but right now I am very paranoid. I thought I was being followed on my way here. I know it isn't true, now, but that's what happens. I find out later. It is the demons. And my brain, you know, it is a schizophrenic brain.

T: Do the meds help?

P: In a way. Sometimes. I don't know. Some bad side effects. I am already too heavy, drugs make it worse, but, well I need to cut down.

The therapist is at first trying to discover the meaning of the delusions, but as he learns how the patient becomes delusional, he wonders about the effect of medication that is aimed at limiting delusions. He then asks about that. In his experience with anti-psychotic medications, they appear to be primarily sedating so that patients with behavioral problems become more manageable, less combative, less restless. It could be that meds here help the patient be "accepting" of his symptoms. However, the therapist has not seen symptom removal, and this patient remains delusional. Indeed, the therapist has seen many patients enter and exit psychiatric hospitals with no alteration in their thinking. The hopeful expectation of such change does not seem to occur very often. Affect does seem to present a different picture because patients frequently become calmer, but at times there is actually a loss of affect and a tendency toward inactivity. His experience is that drugs are primarily sedative, reducing anxiety and activity, but do not alter what he considers to be the "psychotic process," an "unreal reality" which is often harsh and attacks patients in various ways that can involve behavioral problems. There are variations, but a frequent pattern is the suggestion to patients of exaggerated behaviors that lead to interpersonal difficulties. The patients become inappropriate and dysfunctional.

T: I would like you to give this some more thought. I am not sold on your demon theory, but I understand your need for an explanation for these disturbing thoughts and feelings. Often when people sense they know the source of their problems it helps them combat their difficulties. Now schizophrenia is a controversial disorder in that there is a current tendency to stress its possible biological elements, or genetic, or something else other than what might be coming from the social, interpersonal environment, but the truth is we have little certainty about cause or cure.

P: (The patient is quite intelligent, began his career as a health provider, but paranoid delusions caused so much discomfort that he had to stop working. Now he is afraid to work in any environment.) I got that.

T: Now you did all right, were effective, up until you actually began working. Let's even say you were genetically predisposed to become frightened under certain types of pressure, particularly when people are involved who you feel are judging you. You have told me you feel best when you are alone.

P: Yes, I do, but I don't mind my siblings.

T: All right, there are some safe people, perhaps ones who don't judge?

P: Yes, but you are right, I feel most comfortable when I am alone.

T: That includes me as a source of discomfort?

P: Well, yes. I mean I know you are trying to help me, and you do, but I get anxious coming here, like you are going to read my mind.

T: (Laughs.) I wish I could. I imagine you were given ways to be as a child, and adolescent, and your parents were significant models, and some of what went on frightened you, even if the ideas proposed were appropriate, but, somehow, out of reach?

P: I was afraid I would fail. I did well when I was in school, but, really, college, hit the alcohol, the drugs. I was addicted.

T: So, maybe you were having trouble being who you thought you were supposed to be, and at some point you had an occupation, and that made life more scary. The world you were in became a terror for you, and you had to escape, so a part of you, the "demons," took over, but you always seem to be getting criticized by these demons, even though now you don't have to do much.

P: I don't do much, watch TV, oh, and worry, and have delusions and hallucinations, and there are demons, you know.

T: Perhaps there is a devil in all this.

P: Yeah, my father. I can't be around him. I believe he is evil.

T: So, I mean your father seems unaware of how you feel, but none-theless, in a sense with his assistance, you have created this frightening world of punishing demons that makes you feel relatively safe?

P: Could be. (Patient does not seem particularly impressed, but seems relaxed.)

The therapist does considerable shifting of the focus, and the topics, and his approach, as he appears to be searching for what is the most effective mode of oper-ating. He is uncertain, and now that the patient is less anxious the therapist feels more comfortable. The patient has expressed his feelings about his father, so there is a more apparent etiological factor. Of course, this does not mean the patient is about to move toward greater independence. Also, the therapist is aware that some of the directions he has pursued could have been primarily an intellectual exercise to alleviate his anxiety as to the ability to help the patient. The therapist wants the patient to pursue a different, and conceptually better, path for his life but is not sure about what that is or how to try to bring it about. The patient has been hospital-ized, is medicated, knows his thoughts and feelings are distorted from reality, and runs the risk of losing financial support from his father, but finds "another reality."

This therapist has considerable experience with psychotic patients. He usu-ally begins by trying to engage them on what seems to be their terms, a temporary acceptance of their distortions. He has had over time modest success in uncovering what appears to be the purpose of the psychosis, namely a personalized safety with ingredients personalized for the patient. At times he has brought about some shifts to reality acceptance through understanding the contributing motivation and help-ing develop alternatives. In this case, understanding the demon-father connection goes in that direction. However, regressions can and do occur, as these patients are always on the edge of anxiety. The search for what works is especially individual-ized and remains ongoing.

Case 5: Not My Fault

A very helpful point in any talk therapy arrives when the patient takes responsibility for their behavior. It is a welcome transition from "happening to me" to "I am doing it." Once that transition occurs the patient becomes open to the idea that symptoms serve a purpose for the patient. This is the start of an awareness that symptomatic purposing can be costly for the patient. Their restructuring of healthy functioning is damaging rather than protective. Seeing symptom construction as an unsuccessful way to live paves the path to understanding the openness to change, *provided* the patient accepts the responsibility for the symptomatic method being used. If instead, he or she insists they cannot be different, the patient remains relatively static. At issue is finding ways to have patients "buy into" the need for making the change.

The repetition compulsion works against change. It appears to be a "natural" tendency to adhere to thoughts, feelings, and behaviors that result in psychic dis-turbances such as anxiety and depression. The therapist's task is to find ways to eliminate, or at least mitigate, such repetitive patterns. This involves discovering the reasons for the patient's adherence, which requires developmental exploration. Free association provides a fertile field for that, but it is time-consuming, so with the patients depicted here, a focused exploration is used.

Focusing is a relatively personalized process by the therapist, so it is open to countertransference. Of course, whatever the therapist's response or intervention, there is a possibility of countertransference. Sensitivity to that possibility has certainly increased over time, but in a search for what works, oversensitivity could be a problem. We accept the probability of implicit bias but strive to operate in terms of a hierarchy of motivation. That means that we see all the therapist's actions as having a mixture of motivations, some unconscious, but we attempt to build hypotheses based on what we believe is in the patient's best interest. We understand we will not be accurate all of the time.

We propose this formula to the patient: Feel the feeling, experience the thought, ask yourself what the source might be, and guess if necessary. Then, ask yourself, what is this feeling/thought doing for me? Given that symptoms such as anxiety and depression are unpleasant, it usually makes sense to the patient to explore the contradiction that appears. Why be anxious when that anxiety makes one feel worse? Often, the questioning is sufficient to create an interest in changing behavior, but not always.

Such an approach usually requires repetition (working through), given the number of components involved, and at times it is blocked by the patient insisting on a lack of control in creating the symptom. If that is the case, then it is necessary to go back to sorting out the patient's role in having the symptom. However, once that role is established, then the formula can be more successful. In that vein, the following is an example of the difficulties involved.

T: How are you feeling?

P: Anxious, very anxious.

T: What do you think that is about?

P: Well if I knew what it was about I wouldn't feel anxious.

T: Oh, well let's speculate.

P: I shake, my body vibrates, I feel I may fall.

T: If you did fall?

P: It feels like you want me to tell you that I want to feel that way?

T: Do you?

P: You see?

T: I wonder what you would get out of falling?

P: (Sarcastically.) You mean besides a broken leg?

T: (The therapist could explore the patient's resistance, but based on the history of their interaction the therapist feels that would not be effective. There is a tipping point with resistance when it has to be addressed directly or the patient will terminate, but before that, it can be more effective to focus on an issue in a relatively consistent way. The result can be a "neutralization" of resistance where the patient experiences the therapeutic environment as more accepting than confrontational.) No, not so much harm, but some feelings about yourself.

P: I would feel weak.

T: Are there times when you do feel weak?

P: I suppose.

T: Such as?

P: OK, when I get anxious. I mean there is no good reason for me to feel so anxious.

T: (Smiles.) So, a bad reason?

P: (Laughs.) Yeah, a bad reason.

T: Being anxious is unpleasant. It also comes into play when something bothers you.

P: All right, I understand that, but there is nothing that should bother me.

T: Well, for the moment but let's concern ourselves with that "should" part. You did say you feel anxious.

P: Yes, more than I should.

(They both smile at the "should.")

T: Could you describe the anxiety some more, you know, the sensation, thoughts that occur? We can take it from there to get a better idea of what might be going on. (The patient complies, seems more relaxed, more accepting of some agency regarding the symptom.)

Case 6: I Am Addicted

Addiction comes in all shapes, forms, and impacts the person. The presence of a compulsion to do something that is in some way harmful is a widespread problem that society tends to create movements, and at times, laws, to combat. Alcohol and drugs are prominent examples with a focus on abstinence. There is also a tendency to view addiction as a disease, meaning that personal responsibility is shifted from psychodynamic factors, or distorted learning, to willpower. This overlay can still be useful in an integrated approach by supporting the avoidance of the compulsion, but avoidance without understanding the compulsion lessens effectiveness.

P: I have been told by my family physician that my health is at risk if I do not increase my weight.

T: What do you think?

P: I think he does not understand how heavy I am.

T: Would you want to tell me your weight?

P: No, I don't know it. I don't want to know it. I told the doctor not to tell me.

T: Do you have thoughts about why you will not let yourself gain weight?

T: My family is against fat people. My mother is very clear about how bad it is to weigh too much.

T: Is she as thin as you are?

P: No, but she is always watching her weight, and mine.

T: So, she would not like you if you gained weight?

P: She would not say she did not like me, but I know she likes me better than if I was fat.

T: Have you ever been fat?

P: I feel fat now.

T: What does the mirror tell you?

P: I do not look in the mirror.

T: So, who are you pleasing, your mother or you?

P: Both of us.

T: You have been hospitalized because of your weight loss.

P: Well, yes. Maybe I overdid it, though I think at the hospital I was afraid. I know my mother did not want me to be sick.

T: So do you think your feelings about your mother are more complicated than wanting to please her?

P: What do you mean?

T: There are other possibilities. Your mother wants you to be thin, but not to the point of putting yourself at risk?

P: Yes, I don't believe she wants to make me sick.

T: So perhaps you would prefer your mother took a different approach with you?

P: I do wish she was not so fixated on what I eat.

T: Could you tell her that?

P: No, not directly anyway.

T: But you are telling her by the extent to which you are going with your eating, or, not eating.

P: Yes, it does seem that way.

T: By taking it so far you are telling her to be different. You may be angry at her for what you feel she is doing to you?

P: I am, but I don't want to tell her that directly.

T: Not directly, but there is a message in your actions. You are sowing the negative results of how she treats you.

P: Yes, I am.

T: Your approach does not seem to be working. There are other ways to talk with her so that you do not harm yourself. At this point, can you see that?

P: I have to, but it scares me.

T: I know.

This is just the beginning of a slow, lengthy process, but it opens the door to the range of the patient's feelings and how they could be expressed in more productive ways. A useful dynamic in addiction is the awareness that relations can be compulsions and defensive maneuvers to contain undesirable feelings, usually aggression, that cause harm to the patient as well as others while avoiding direct expression of feelings. Although these are often hostile feelings, the compulsion defense is not that successful because it antagonizes others anyway. However, the addicted person is caught up in what they view as their own needed protection and the chemical properties of any used substance facilitate the continued use. Also, classifying certain compulsions as diseases can have the effect of "inevitability" where the patient assumes the symptoms have to be overpowering and can limit motivation to change. The conception described here is that a psychodynamic explanation is *one possibility* that merits consideration among many possible explanations for addiction.

Case 7: No Respect

The patient finds himself in what appears to be an untenable situation. His wife and adult children find it difficult to interact with him and avoid interaction. They have all told him that he does not discuss but argues and attacks them verbally when any discussion is attempted. At this point the children are not talking to him and his wife is limiting their contact. He is coming to therapy at their urging because they are telling him he needs to change.

P: I don't know what is going on with them. I have been a good husband, provider, caretaker, but they don't want to talk to me.

T: They are avoiding you?

P: Every time I try to talk to one of them, after a few minutes, it is over.

T: So, with your wife with whom you live, she does not talk to you?

P: I try to get her to talk, to show me some concern, some warmth, but after a few minutes she tells me she has to go.

T: Do you think it is what you are talking about, or more the way you are talking? (The patient was talking in an increasingly loud and assertive manner and appeared to be getting agitated.)

P: What do you mean?

T: Is it the way that you talk to her?

P: (Speaking in an angry tone.) How should I talk to her? She is my wife. She should listen.

T: You seem angry.

P: I am angry. She should listen to me. You should listen to me.

T: I am listening and I hear anger.

P: You do, do you? Well of course I am angry. I should be angry. She wants everything her way, forget about me, but she wouldn't have a thing if it wasn't for me. She is cold, she is cruel, she's impossible.

T: You are angry with me. Why is that?

P: Of course, you will agree with her, take her side. (Patient is now pacing around the room.)

T: Could you sit down so that we can talk?

P: (Patient sits.) What do you want to talk about?

T: You said your wife leaves you when you want to talk. It just seemed as if you were leaving me.

P: I'm sitting. Go ahead, talk.

T: Perhaps you are annoyed at having to be here when the people who are annoying you are not here.

P: Yeah, ok. I mean, it isn't you.

T: Here is the issue. The people you want to spend time with are avoiding you because of how you talk to them. In essence, the problem is your style.

P: So I said a few hostile things. It is how I get. They all know that. It is me when I get angry.

T: Sounds like that is often and they have had enough.

P: Yeah, well too bad. Let them act different.

T: I understand, you are the father and you want respect, but your method for getting it is not working.

P: So, too bad for them.

T: I am afraid it is too bad for you.

P: You are on their side.

T: I want you to get what you want. I understand how you feel that you have already earned it by your support of the family, but they appear not to agree.

P: They should agree.

T: This is not about what they should do, but what will work.

P: Listen to me. You don't seem to get that I am right and they are wrong.

T: Consider this, that your strength lies in your ability to find a way to talk to your family that enables them to listen.

P: You mean they don't have to change, but I do.

T: It seems so.

P: All right, I will be quiet for a while, but not for long.

This type of conversation, specifics varying, is repeated for many sessions. The patient's self-esteem is dependent on feeling loved and respected by his family in very concrete expressions of gratitude that are not forthcoming. Instead, they are indicating that they are currently "putting up with him." They see him as emotionally abusive while he denies that and sees himself as having made their lives comfortable. They feel they have survived and thrived despite him, while he feels it is because of him. He tries threatening them, but they are not afraid. They want to get along with him, but for this to happen they indicate that he has to change. Based on the therapist's interactions with the patient, he views the patient as the one with the problem, and that the patient does need to change his manner and behavior. He also believes that the patient could do that if the patient viewed the ability to adapt to change as a strength. His focus needs to be on "what works," rather than what the patient thinks is "right." At first glance this may seem unlikely to happen, but it is also clear to the therapist that the patient wants to preserve the family unit, so he continues to work with that as the desired outcome.

This case is also an opportunity to look at how the basic psychoanalytic concept of neutrality can be involved in integrative work. Explored in detail recently by Lafarge (2022), neutrality is a concept whose meaning has shifted with the evolution of psychoanalysis which has a basic consistent purpose. It was intended to foster mental freedom for the patient by creating a state of mind of non-directedness. The situation designed to provide the most direct route to the patient's unconscious that would be displayed was free association. In integrative therapy associations are limited and focused, so neutrality is also limited. The therapist wants the patient to pursue a particular line of thinking and feeling, an intersubjective one that involves recognition of his own vulnerability and the need to explore and incorporate a more sensitive and practical approach to his relationship with his family. Integrative work is directed neutrality, the direction being material that is important to the resolution of the patient's difficulties. However, direction is obtained from the patient so the therapist is neutral in terms of personal framing elements. These refer to social beliefs and issues, such as internal sexism, racism, theoretical models, and personal preferences for the therapist's current listening mode.

Case 8: Sort of True

This patient had been married for some time but was relatively inexperienced sexually before that. Now, as a single person again he is very concerned about the meaning of sexuality in a relationship. His self-image was dependent on constant reassurance from his partner, and he operated in a relatively traditional manner. She was very devoted to him, and her loss has resulted in significant loneliness and a search for a person to alleviate his anxiety and make him feel safe again. The woman he is now with also lost her partner but has had some subsequent relationships and appears to have had considerable sexual experience.

P: When I met her, well, she admitted she was experienced.

T: How did that make you feel?

P: I didn't like it, but I like her. I suppose I was jealous, or I was afraid she would find somebody else, and I didn't ask for the details. (Pauses.)

T: And now?

P: We were out with a couple of her girlfriends and I think they kind of forgot I was there, or they were trying to tell me something, or they didn't care, I don't know, but they were fooling around making references to the guys that she had been involved with, but not critical, more like how she attracts all these men, gets them to be really involved with her.

T: They forgot you were there?

P: I know, not really. I think they were trying to get across to me how she is, you know, lucky me, look how all these guys went for her.

T: Do you feel lucky?

P: Not really, no, I felt jealous, angry at her. I mean, she wasn't embarrassed or anything. More like proud.

T: And?

P: So, later, when were alone, I told her it bothered me. She laughed it off, said I was jealous.

T: Sounds like you were upset.

P: I am. I feel like she lied to me, although I never really asked, like, how many?

T: So she did not really lie?

P: No, but that doesn't matter so much. I don't like that she slept with other men. I do feel like I can't trust her, and also, maybe they were better than me.

T: She wants you now.

P: Yes, but I can't seem to let it go. I keep bringing it up to her. She tells me, forget about it. It didn't mean anything. She thinks I am insecure.

T: Is that how you feel?

P: Yes, insecure. I mean, I don't see myself as a great lover or anything. Sometimes I have trouble. I have not slept with many women.

T: She's experienced, you are not, but she wants you.

P: True, but how can I trust her, and I really like her, but knowing this, I mean am I just another guy she sleeps with?

T: Well, you are both older, been married and divorced. It does seem you both could be experienced?

P: Well, she is way ahead of me apparently. Look, I don't want to obsess about it, but I do.

T: You said you like her?

P: Yes, very much, but I mean, is she some kind of slut?

T: Strong word. Does sexual experience equate automatically with her being unfaithful to you?

P: Sounds like you are trying to convince me it is not that important?

T: I don't see why it has to be, given that you really like her.

P: You don't think it matters?

T: It does matter to you, but. . . . (Therapist pauses.)

P: Because I am insecure.

T: I don't think it has to remain a problem, and yes, your insecurity, and your different sexual history, are having an effect. I don't know how trustworthy she is, but she seems to want you now, and you wanted her.

P: I still want her. I mean, I have been looking for a while and she is it, or is she?

T: Well, she told you she was experienced and she could have been defensive when her girlfriends brought it up, but she wasn't, so she seems all right with her past. I don't know how she will be in the future, but you know, having an experienced partner could be helpful to you given your performance concerns.

P: She is patient, never critical about how I am sexually, but once again, it feels like you are trying to talk me into trusting her.

T: My feelings are showing. Of course, I am not you. Still, her past sexual behavior does not equate to potential unfaithfulness.

P: I think I get it. I don't like to face the fact that I am so insecure. I mean, I am old enough now, and been around, so why am I so afraid of what might happen?

T: Now that you see the issue that is bothering you with more clarity? (Pauses.)

P: (Laughs.) I know, we can explore it.

This particular segment covers several issues; the therapist's countertransference which suggests personal experience with sexual behavior as well as a more liberal attitude than the patient's, and the patient's personal issues regarding self-esteem, sexuality, and trust. There is an attempt to "correct" the patient's thinking and feeling, and there is also some exploration of the patient's development that is reflected in his insecurity and distrust. The patient is left to decide for himself what he wants to do about the relationship. The "nudge" from the therapist is primarily in the direction of examining the patient's insecurity, though there is an implication that the patient can benefit from continuing his relationship with the woman.

Case 9: The Dream

This patient reports dreams frequently but usually indicates that he does not remember the content. This time the dream was recalled.

> P: I had a dream. I was walking along on a street in a city, probably New York City, and there was an accident at the crosswalk. People were pushing and shoving others to see what was happening, and somebody shoved me, and I cried out, and I said, it is you, Pud, and that's all I recall.
>
> T: What are your thoughts?
>
> P: At first, I thought, the city scares me, no walking there, I would be afraid just to be there. The accident, I suppose I would expect that too, the city is dangerous and people are pushy, more hurtful than helpful.
>
> T: Does the "dangerous city" with its "accidents" and "hurtful people" include a specific place?
>
> P: You mean, other than New York City?
>
> T: Yes, some other setting.
>
> P: (Smiles.) Like here, like therapy maybe?
>
> T: Could be.
>
> P: All right, lately I have been feeling pressure here, like you were pushing me.
>
> T: So, the "accident" could happen, you could be in some danger?
>
> P: You could be getting me to talk about something I don't want to talk about because it will hurt me, so you are like everybody else, push, shove, make me fall. In fact, you were there, in the dream you were there. I saw you.
>
> T: "Pud"?
>
> P: Yes, puddle, and I will drown and you will just swim away.
>
> T: (Thinks puddle is a stretch to drown, or to swim in, but puddle could expand to pool. However, the therapist associated Pud to Bud, and to feel helpful, and wants to be seen that way by the patient, but realizes that was not the patient's perception.) Perhaps I wanted to get away too.
>
> P: (Surprised.) Well, in the dream, the push, puddle, you seemed hostile.
>
> T: Or afraid of the big city like you, maybe sensing both of us were in dangerous territory. Sounds like Pud needs to get Mud, slow down. I need to be patient, walk with you, not push.
>
> P: And watch where we are walking.

This is one way to use countertransference. The material lends itself to further interpretation. The fact that the patient saw the therapist in the dream is not an automatic signifier that the dream is about the therapy or the therapist's actions. The therapist could be a substitute for another significant person in the patient's life. Other parts of the dream suggest other possibilities. Of particular interest is what the patient wants to avoid. Also, the therapist is being told to be helpful, but not push. The patient might be falling as a message for the need for immediate help. It also could be that the patient does feel close enough to the therapist to ask for it via the dream, a "do more" message, not just a "don't push." Also, it would be useful for the therapist to explore personal feelings regarding being pictured as a "pushy person in a crowd." As with all dreams, numerous interpretations are possible.

When It Does Not Work

The material presented thus far was in support of an integrative method that facilitates treatment. However, the avoidance of therapy by many who could use it is high, as is the drop-out rate, one to two sessions. While insurance providers like brief therapy they do not advocate either avoidance or very brief treatment. We let all our patients know that psychotherapy is usually a lengthy process and that consistent attendance and commitment to the process are vital for therapy to be successful. Also, we are realistic with patients concerning the limits of our "curative" possibilities. There is a "good fit" issue, meaning that our efforts are not always suitable from the patient's viewpoint.

Often that is due to countertransference issues, some of which, in retrospect, we could have avoided. In general, it appears that therapists get in more trouble from what they do say, as interpretations, comments, or the use of a hard word, such as "depressed," compared to "down," rather than what they do not. However, analysts in particular have been criticized for their silence and apparent distance while they are attempting to be very attentive and listen.

It appears that there are "readiness" and "compatibility" factors that play a significant role for patients. These are not reflective of the quality of the psychotherapy being offered. A few patients who leave therapy because the office was too dark are at variance with those who left because it was too bright, and both sets are just not ready for therapy although they may be needed. As therapists we do have to accept the probability that some people are just not going to accept our best efforts, but we must keep giving our best efforts.

The Crooked Path of Effectiveness

Intersectionality

Intersectionality describes the nature of social categories that are applied most often to a designated group that involves overlapping systems, such as people who are Black and poor. Although we will discuss other issues of intersectionality in later chapters, our focus here is on psychotherapy, so the categorical groups are methodology and results. As noted in previous chapters, treatment methods have shifted in preference over time, so although psychodynamic was once dominant, it has now been replaced by behavioral. Each approach claimed to have the answer, but, as also noted, mental health treatment remains relatively ineffective. Psychoanalysis based its evidence primarily on the faith of both therapist and patient while behavioral therapies based their belief on suspect evidence. At the moment, behavioral approaches have gained the most acceptance. The intersectionality now discriminates against psychoanalysis that it is too lengthy, too expensive.

Intersectionality, the inevitable interlock of time, money, and limited evidence, creates a negative view of psychoanalysis. Of course, it can be applied to positive related stacking, but the more frequent application is to a negative view of a category, usually a broad one, such as race, class, or gender, that is inaccurate and harmful to both individuals and society in some fashion. For example, in the mental health field consider the possibility that drugs could be touted as the "cure all," replacing talk therapy as the method of effectiveness. The intersectionality is conceptual, namely drug therapy and effectiveness, are equated and talk therapy is markedly disadvantaged. Now up to this point that has not happened because drug compliance requires verbal persuasion, drugs have limited effectiveness, and side effects are sufficient to keep that possibility at bay, but it is a thought. The problem with intersectionality is not the overlap, but how the interconnectedness may automatically be used in a discriminating fashion, namely a "pile-on effect" that when examined more closely is unwarranted.

There are tempting reasons to use the overlap in a distorted manner. In mental health treatment, drugs are easier and simpler to use than talk therapy. In the talk therapy field behavioral treatment is less expensive, requires less training, and takes less time, but these apparent advantages are not automatically linked to effectiveness. Ease, simplicity, or cost reduction should not be the criteria for usage. The complexity of mental illness, and even more basic, the complexity of human functioning, are powerful attestations for life-cycle treatment possibilities for many people and for many problems. It is important to keep this in mind when recognizing the possibility of intersectionality where it would be inaccurate to equate longer duration and cost with ineffectiveness.

Also, the motivation of providers to choose their roles, including the pharmaceutical industry and the numerous health providers, particularly managed care, are involved in a very large industry with a vested interest in financial reward. We like to believe that the industry has a heart that goes beyond, or even before, self-interest. As a result, we have to avoid creating an intersectional trap under the guise of having found "the answer." It is not a singular solution, nor will it be. Integration, with all its diffusion, is the more likely effective solution.

Integration

An integrative model for psychotherapy requires a different training approach than what is used currently. Now psychotherapy training is relatively specialized, essentially limited by the theoretical preferences of the trainers. Psychoanalysts teach psychoanalytic approaches, of which there are many, and behavioral therapists teach behavioral techniques, and there are a variety of mental health counselors, nurses and social workers, and psychiatrists who have very limited psychotherapy training. Integration of the techniques is rare, and these disciplines tend to be more competitive than supportive of each other. It would be unusual to find a provider who had been trained in an integrated model, so complicated intersectionality prevails.

In terms of overall training for the treatment of mental illness, psychiatry is lengthy but relies heavily on the use of drugs. Behavior therapy training tends to be brief and in line with the actual practice of the therapy and is talk therapy. Psychoanalysis is by far the most extensive psychotherapy training but is usually influenced heavily by a particular analytic theory. There has also been a trend toward specializing in trauma therapy, or specific disorders such as phobias, compulsions, or addictions, which tends to obscure the frequent comorbidity as well as the limitations involved in describing psychiatric disorders. Psychoanalysis appears to be the only therapy that requires the trainees to be in therapy themselves. Also, psychoanalysts are more focused on personality reconstruction while behavior therapists emphasize symptom alleviation, so the latter appear more specialized.

Theories abound as to the etiologies as well as the treatments. The terms "mental health" and "mental illness" are used as though they had precise meanings for all involved, which they often do not. For example, anxiety can be considered a mental illness, for example, generalized anxiety disorder, when it reaches a certain level of discomfort for a person, but that level is a variable viewed subjectively by the person with the anxiety. Also, the very process of living has stresses that can be expected to result in anxiety, and this is also true for depression. Usually, the need for help arises when feelings, thoughts, or behavior disrupt a person's functioning to a degree that they, or others around them, feel is significant. That, too, is a variable, person and environment-dependent. All this is noted to emphasize the "inexactness" of the field, starting with who are to be categorized as patients.

Although psychoanalysis has fallen out of favor, and has significant limitations, it still provides an opportunity not available elsewhere for a person to essentially evaluate themselves and open themselves to scrutiny psychologically by therapists who are trained to enable such a process. Given that psychoanalytic training is the most extensive and detailed regarding personality structure and development, and we have a lot of experience with it, we will use that as a model to work from in developing more integrative possibilities to meet current mental health concerns.

Some Considerations

In most instances, other than psychoanalytic field theory, psychoanalytic training has kept a distance from the social environment. However, the construction of a mental health delivery system is a complex social endeavor. It involves recognition of the provider's identity as part of a social structure that affects the existence and role of the provider. The complexity of analysts as mental health providers within a system that depends on being integrated has been avoided by picturing the analyst as a neutral observer. The original connection of psychoanalysis to health issues seems to be a forgotten background as the theorizing moved in the direction of creating theories of the mind. Of course, such theories are of interest to society, and at one point people were quite psychoanalytic-minded, but that is no longer the case. For present relevance, there has to be a recognition that we are part of the health delivery system, and that system has its own demands. Psychoanalytic training has to become more socially sophisticated.

There is behavior that is disruptive to society, and that behavior is not always accompanied by logical explanation, and that behavior is often classified as mental illness, with the absence of such behavior as mental health. People look for the presence of ethics in a society that will guarantee behavior by most of the population that provides for the comfort and happiness of most people. Rules are created as a framework for behavior and each society develops means of enforcement. Analysts live and work in society, and the work we are tasked with doing is dealing with the mentally ill, and that takes in a lot of people that were not the usual analytic patients, such as addicts, homeless, severely disturbed, and subjects of discrimination. Also, society created an unexpected entity for us called managed care. Psychoanalytic training just did not stay attuned to shifts in society that would affect what we do and as a result, we have to tune in now and work with the flow. Thus, analytic training needs social consciousness and learning how to be actively involved in how society functions, as well as considering how other nations function.

The variance involved in learning this is extensive. In a democratic society there is more flexibility in behavior than in an autocratic one, but democracy is not an automatic indicator of mental health. If leaders are elected, people are not personally safer than under authoritarian leaders. Rebellions are not an automatic sign of mental health, because it depends on what happens to the rebels, their cause, and the outcome of the rebellion. A major issue is the maintenance of emotional stability in an environment that makes that difficult. Freedom of expression seems more likely than constraint, but many people have to learn to develop an emotional balance under difficult circumstances. Mental health and illness are social concepts, basically contextual.

There are diagnostic criteria for mental illness, but they are dependent primarily on how people view themselves and present themselves to others rather than a diagnostic tool, such as testing blood. If a person feels anxious to the point that it limits their functioning, then the person may see himself as having a mental illness problem. If a person bothers others sufficiently, such as engaging in an unprovoked physical attack, that person will also be considered to have a mental illness problem. As therapists we tend to accept the mental illness category based on people presenting themselves to us with a stated emotional problem, such as anxiety, or society giving us the people because they harmed themselves or others. Also, part of the context is that we try to help people who have problems in living, such as being indecisive, shy, or lonely, and it can be a stretch to call the problem mental illness, but these issues can cause anxiety and depression. Given the turbulent state of world affairs, it appears that mental illness is rampant at the same time that so many people are asking for emotional peace, all of which emphasize the importance of improving the mental health delivery systems.

Considering the social, political, and economic influences on both diagnosing and treating the problems of living and the adjective "complex" seems an understatement. At present we have an evolving, struggling treatment system with a large variety of treatments and helpers with a variety of training, skill, and experience. In one sense, it is fascinating that we fare as well as we do, but it is not that adequate and there is plenty of room for improvement. An effective mental health system needs to become much more of a priority for our society than it is.

Our initial premise is that everybody has the right to have effective health care and that society must make that possible. This country flirts with that possibility through the existing entitlements that have been developed, such as Social Security, Medicare, and Medicaid, and people welcome these programs. These have come about because they are both needed and desired by the majority of people. These programs came about slowly, given that they involve intersectionality, namely socialism and control, in a democracy that prizes freedom. Extending this approach certainly will bring problems. As an example, the intricacies and systemic issues of Medicare are enormous, but not insurmountable. Our society is more likely to prosper if it is at maximum health, so it is a reasonable direction to contemplate. It appears accurate to describe our country as a socialized democracy in which the competitive aspect is very much alive. Can we then not reasonably ask that all people be allowed to be healthy?

We believe that society should provide the necessities of life to all its members, and we readily admit there is self-interest and healthy narcissism involved in that belief. To preserve the elements of competition there will undoubtedly be debates as to what those necessities are. As a start we offer food, shelter, clothing, and health care, all of which rely on economic support, which will move the argument to how that support is to be provided. Our current system is a mixture of private and public financing, and for health care, it is a mixture of public, insurance through employers, and out-of-pocket payment. The last alternative is by far the least frequent and used primarily by affluent people. The employer-connected insurance has become restrictive in its managed-care controls. The result is a limited supply of health care possibilities. It appears that a Medicare-for-all type approach is the most likely to make health care available to all that is needed. That brings up both how it gets financed and how it gets administered. We do not consider ourselves experts in this regard and understand that it will be ultimately a political decision. We do have an opinion, which is that all health providers push for a measure that improves better access to health providers than the existing systems, and in so doing they weigh in on the particulars so that decisions about type, frequency, and duration of treatment returns to the province of patients and providers as well as reasonable fees. Regarding costs being appropriate, that could mean cuts for some providers and increases for others. As far as reasonable goes, during the COVID-19 emergency periods, psychotherapy fees were increased by Medicare, but once the "emergency" period passed they were cut back, and a further step was taken to reduce them for 2023 below what they had been the previous year, which at best seemed disingenuous. Also, while Medicare has psychotherapy fees based on time spent with the patient, they much prefer therapists use the 45-minute session than the 50, the former being cheaper, although there is certainly no evidence that giving patients less time improves their mental health. These are just some examples that illustrate specific management problems and show the need for provider involvement.

Increasing an entitlement, for example, Medicare for all, does involve an acceptance of wealth redistribution because it would have to involve taxation. It means that people who worked diligently to amass wealth would be paying for treatment for less wealthy people, and in many cases, poor. This raises the possibility of exploring a motivational shift. This country has long been known as the land of opportunity, the phrase appealing to many as an economic opportunity. We offer for consideration that the opportunity to thrive includes the opportunity to help those who have not been able to thrive to a sufficient degree to meet their basic needs, health care being prominent as a necessity. Raising social consciousness in this regard could be a mission for all possible training as well as a very desirable social vision.

Psychoanalytic Training

The providers of mental health services are numerous and diverse and vary in the extensiveness of their training, which results in segmented services, namely people doing what they have been trained to do. That can be useful, but an important feature of being a provider in all that diversity is to stay within the level of competence acquired. Intersectionality at times prevails unfortunately in that one discipline will attempt to exclude another based on the assumption of greater competence. Psychiatry has moved in the direction of medication and now offers limited training in psychotherapy. Psychology and other disciplines such as social work and counseling have moved in the direction of behavioral approaches. Psychoanalysis has embraced pluralism but made the choices exclusive. There is a divisiveness to all this which is not helpful in the provision of effective mental health services. Our reaction is to emphasize the need for integrative therapy, of which at the moment, there is very little.

Given that psychoanalytic training is the most extensive of the talk therapies, and that many of its concepts are used in other therapies, we will consider how that can be made flexible and integrative. A general suggestion is that exposure to behavioral approaches should be made available. In addition, pluralism should be expansive and thorough. Providers should also be familiar with psychiatric medication. The results, which could hold for all disciplines, is a broad-based approach providing effective exposure to what is available for the treatment of mental disorders. In addition, there is a societal concern with implicit basis, systemic racism, and the existence of feelings that may be unconscious, but nonetheless are getting expressed. This needs to be explored as part of understanding countertransference (Shah, 2020).

The Clinical Moments Project (Tuch & Kuttnauer, 2018) provides refreshing transparency into psychoanalytic training in the presentation and discussion of specific clinical incidents that proved to be difficult for therapists. The incidents are described in greater detail than we are including, the problems are indicated to commentators, who respond, and the subsequent actions of the therapists are noted. We will discuss some of this material in a relatively concise manner and indicate how it could be reacted to using an integrated approach.

The first case involves a man who is anxious about being proven wrong and is resistant to treatment. At this point in the therapy his attendance is irregular based on his circumstances, and in the sessions, he tends to make use of slips of the tongue that could be open to interpretation. Given the fragility of the therapeutic alliance the therapist is trying to decide whether or not to interpret. The patient has described a tendency on his part to be "grabby," and then he takes that back. The "grabby" comment could be viewed as an example of the underlying defense and underlying anxiety about an idea that was expressed. Pointing out the slip could make the patient anxious but being silent misses an opportunity for him to understand more about himself. A basic issue is finding out what is making the patient anxious. He is afraid of being inappropriate. One suggested possibility would be to ask the patient what his "grabby" thought might be making him anxious, emphasizing an interpretive approach.

A different viewpoint would be a focus on the patient-therapist relational experience. If the therapist focuses on what the patient said, and in turn, what he indicated he did not want to say, there is an implication of wrongness on the patient's part that could increase his resistance. Instead, another suggestion was to inquire about the patient's apparent anxiety in the therapist-patient interaction. This can be seen as facilitating an awareness of the patient's dominant pattern of self-organization.

Both of the comments, suggested by other therapists looking at the case, illustrate the issue of the need to integrate interpersonal and intrapsychic possibilities that are available in a psychoanalytic conceptualization. Integration is not suggested. Instead, they each suggest going one way, which highlights the need to teach both approaches, be aware of both dimensions, and consider how to integrate them.

The patient appears both anxious and ambivalent, so both issues need to be addressed to facilitate the progression of treatment. The actual therapist in this case decided to focus on the patient's anxiety, allowing for a mutual recognition of the anxiety and the therapists reported that it appeared to mitigate the ambivalence. The patient's use of undoing was noted as an example of anxiety, and directly addressing it seemed to provide both relief for the patient (and probably for the therapist as well). This appears to be integrative, providing both symptom relief and support for the therapeutic alliance. Interpretation is at the level of noting a reaction as a sign of anxiety and moving towards understanding the reason for the reaction. This seems appropriate at this point in the therapy and is carried out without noting the patient's "mistake" as a way of avoiding increasing his anxiety.

In a different case the therapist is trying to decide on the most appropriate interpretation to use. One commentator indicates that there is no "right way," a very useful comment that supports the reality of the many possibilities available. A problem in training is the tendency to offer a particular method as if it is the *only* way to do things properly, even if other ways may be mentioned. It is increasingly obvious that there are multiple ways to address a problem and the therapist is tasked with finding the way that *works* because each patient is likely to require different interventions. An issue that arises in this case is the type of interpretation, transferential or extra-transferential. Transferential refers to a direct reference by the therapist to her influence, but this distinction is often compromised with the therapy appearing as a complete representation of the patient's inner life. Also, in this case the actual therapist indicates an awareness of what she considers empathic failures on her part.

In one instance, she suggested the patient was disappointed with her, which the patient denied and switched topics. The therapist apparently did not like that and became distracted, which the patient noticed, expressed annoyance, and raised doubts about continuing in therapy. How that was resolved was not indicated, but the therapy continued. Disinterest occurs again, although again the therapy continues, raising the question of how the empathic failures get resolved. For example, what is the therapist's issue with this patient? That is not clear, so conjecture is that the problem lies in the therapist's expectations. What the patient says, or does not say means something, and that is supposed to interest the therapist. However, if the therapist wants a particular response or focus from the patient and does not get it, the therapist might react negatively. There may be times when the therapist does not want the patient to know how she is reacting, and there may be other times when the therapist would want the patient to know the expectations, disappointment by the therapist, and have a discussion about the reaction. It seems in this case that the patient could pick up disinterest by the therapist, even react to it, but not discuss it yet continue with treatment as though there had been no rupture, and the therapist went along as well.

The therapist also reported another instance in which the therapist felt a lack of attunement concerning the patient's feelings, although the patient moved on quickly, determined to keep up the appearance of positive transference. The most recent issue was about the interpretation of a dream. The therapist was wondering whether she should focus interpretation on what appeared to be a rupture in the therapy, or not. One commentator suggested the therapist does not have to be so careful about saying the right thing, which seems quite accurate given the patient's tendency to move on, no matter what the therapist does. Clearly there could be a limit to the patient's tolerance, so the suggestion was likely a general one that happens to be supported in this particular case by the patient's behavior.

Another commentator indicated that exploration that focuses on the patient's inability to accept imperfections (a self-described trait of the patient) does not explain why she feels as she does. A comment is also made that corrective experience could be applied to help her accept disappointment but would not change her belief in the threat of the lack of perfection. Emphasis is given to using the transference to facilitate the patient's understanding of her cause for concern. The interpretation issue is the possibility of both helping the patient to accept the reality of relationships and having her understand the reasons for her difficulty in accepting limitations. There appears to be tension between the patient and the therapist. They seem to struggle, with the patient turning away negative feelings because she feels she has to keep a positive view of the therapist. In contrast, the therapist at times has contrary feelings, and for significant reasons as far as the therapist is concerned, though what they are was not clear in the description provided. Exploration of their relationship, particularly how it proceeds, seems a useful way toward better understanding and more comfortable behavior. The therapist appears aware of the times when attunement is inaccurate or lacking, and at this point seems particularly concerned that it not be repeated. However, while the patient initially reacts to these events with negative reactions, she quickly presents a positive transferential picture. It would seem useful to explore the negative transference rather than seeming to let the patient cover it. So, while there may not be one right thing to say, there does seem to be a procedure that would be helpful, and integrative.

Also, one commentator indicated that corrective experience would help her accept disappointment but would not change her belief in the threat of imperfection. It is not clear if that procedure was ruled out because it was considered behavioral and/or because it would alter the transference in being more authoritarian. However, given that it is part of a depth-oriented therapy and that co-construction is considered acceptable, it would seem useful. A relational approach already changes the transference dynamic, given that it is aimed at reducing the authoritarian atmosphere of traditional analysis. Also, this patient persists in seeing the therapist in a positive manner, regardless of what the therapist has been doing, so it is unlikely to have created a change in the patient's view of the therapist. It does seem that transference is very persistent in its quality for patients and is unlikely to be altered by integrative procedures.

A third case involves a man who came into therapy because he was depressed. He had two previous treatments and left both because he considered them ineffective. He described his current life as pleasant, although he said his wife disagreed, and stated he had a happy childhood. However, after the patient elaborated on his childhood, the therapist had a different impression. Subsequently, it became apparent to the patient that he had experienced a difficult, lonely early development, and he seemed to accept that view. However, when the therapist at some point raised the possibility that early feelings of bitterness and sadness could be present in his current life, he became angry and denied current problems. He developed paranoid rage that dominated the sessions, but the therapist continued to link current feelings with childhood experiences. At some point the patient threatened to quit if the therapist continued with this approach. The question for the therapist was, should he confront the paranoid fears, or avoid what the patient did not want discussed?

One commentator suggested that the analyst move away from trying to analyze early experiences and focus on the current relationship with the patient. The other commentator suggested offering alternative contexts, such as the repetition of leaving therapy, or the good therapist having become the bad therapist. Both suggestions put the focus on transference and countertransference.

The patient described a dream in the next session in which he was very afraid. It appears no attempt was made to have the patient interpret the dream. Instead, the therapist indicated the dream represented a part of the patient that he feared and was burying. He also told the patient that the patient was trying to silence him as well. The patient responded by saying that there was a real threat that the therapist did not see, but the patient did not repeat the threat to quit therapy. In the next session the patient reported having had the same dream again, and now he said the therapist might be correct. The therapy continued and it is reported that their "crisis" was subsequently discussed. It would seem appropriate to have had the patient indicate what he thought the dream was about, but given their difficulties, the therapist found a way to move on by using it to support his view of the patient's issues, and it worked. Issues that may have been involved in the dream that might have been revealed by the patient can be addressed later. In one sense the therapist was integrative, switching his approach to direct suggestion, while in another he stayed with the same context of establishing the impact of early experience.

What is apparent in this case, as well as in the previous ones, is that a lot goes on between the patients and the therapists that can be difficult to discuss. It also seems that the therapists are prone to focus on interpretation of the patients' experiences rather than the interpersonal aspects of the therapy. There is a reliance on sufficient positive transference that the therapy is eased through potential times of discomfort by having negative transference bypassed. While this keeps the therapy going and can both make the therapist more comfortable and provide positive effects for the patients, it leaves a lot of feelings, particularly negative ones, unrecognized and unresolved. It suggests that therapists are theory-bound to an approach emphasized in their training, namely interpretation as a therapeutic goal. At the same time, the institute invited the commentators there, and the commentators tend to point out the lack of interpersonal exploration, so it may be that some shift is happening in the training. The first integration that is suggested here is within the pluralism of psychoanalytic approaches. It certainly would be a more expansive experience for patients and therapists, but it seems blocked by an awareness of countertransference that indicates a strong need to keep the patients in therapy. Better use could be made of that awareness.

The issue has to be that therapy is supposed to be what works for the patient. The integrative approach indicates that the focus is on the patient's satisfaction, but that does not mean avoidance of discussing tensions between the participants, particularly when patients are threatening to leave. The therapist does have to decide what is appropriate, and it is apparent in the cases mentioned that some material is excluded that could be pertinent. However, it is certainly possible that these samples reflect timing and a judgment that the issues would be more productive if discussed when the therapeutic alliance felt stronger. The question, which has to be answered in the clinical situation, is, has the patient been helped, and that involves timing, omissions, and inclusions? What has been described is used here to indicate both what was carried out and what could have been in addition, or in place of what did occur.

Disruptions

For therapy to be client-centered it has to produce the results desired by the patient. During the process there are likely to be times when the patient disagrees or is unhappy with the therapist regarding the procedure, such as the topics to be explored, interpretations, the therapist's attitude, the atmosphere being created, or some type of negative transference. So, the question arises as to the degree that the process is to be controlled by the therapist. In traditional analysis the analyst fits into a more authoritative role, apparently neutral but usually the ultimate interpreter. Most behavioral methods are structured by the therapist. Relational approaches emphasize co-construction, but the therapist is usually the ultimate influencer. In the cases described, the influence was such that the patients reacted by threatening to leave, and the therapists had to find ways to keep the procedure intact.

As a result, therapists have to consider the impact of negative transference that can reach such intensity that some patients do terminate. The therapist is expected to be the expert in determining the procedure, and enacting it, so the patient has to accept enough to form a therapeutic alliance. Effective procedure requires mutual participation, in that sense, co-construction. So, if the therapist believes certain topics need to be discussed for the therapy to work, but the patient disagrees, accommodations need to be made. This means the therapist needs to provide a logic for the approach that allows the patient to continue. In terms of participation, the patient is in control, and if a therapist does not allow for this, then there will be trouble. The probability is that if the therapist is insistent on an approach, a lot will be missed if the therapy continues. It is more effective to be open to shifts, to have a fluid sensibility, and avoid being tethered to theory or procedure. Therapists can be flexible, indicate what they think is the appropriate course, but take the view that this is where the person wants to be now, so let us be there and see what happens later.

Most current therapies are time-limited, so although continued therapy could be productive, in many cases the ideal coverage may not be possible. The issue for therapists is to be able to distinguish between avoidances that are necessary at certain points because of circumstances and avoidances that could be avoided, and would limit therapeutic results, but are patient-created and are resistances. At times it is necessary to use a stop-restart approach based on the patient's reactions. The patient is the ultimate decider, though the therapist needs to be comfortable with the agreed-upon course of therapy. All patients are not experienced by therapists with the same degree of interest and concern, so that means there is shifting countertransference in terms of whom is appealing to work with, which in turn affects the procedure. Similar variations are likely to be found in patients, where some therapists are a "pass-through"; others are "life-savers." The best arrangement, not hard to figure, is a "good match."

Further Comments

In the Clinical Moments Project with numerous commentators, expectations as to emphasis were varied. One possibility was giving priority to interaction aimed at providing insight and having that be at an emotional level. Therapists with this view felt transference interpretation was essential and was viewed as a way to actualize patients' core issues and involve an intrapsychic emphasis. Others disagreed about the value of transference interpretation and insight. The probability is that there are multiple viewpoints as to the conduct of therapy, and that they all can work to some degree, some better than others depending on the patient. While it is certainly difficult to learn the many possibilities effectively, it is important to be aware of them. Training institutes can be most effective by providing extensive exposure. The emphasis needs to be on learning what works, with therapists always looking to improve with that in mind. Therapists will likely have favorites, existing pluralism making that clear, but hopefully their interest represents demonstrated effectiveness.

Tuch and Kuttnauer (2018) describe some possibilities, starting with listening to the patient and attending to behavior that seems to represent underlying factors. Another possibility is repairing deficits and aiding patients to satisfy self-object needs. Of particular interest, and moving markedly in an integrative direction, is an emphasis, not on *what* to consider, but on *how* to engage the patient (Nicoli & Bolognini, 2022). This approach is pluralistic with psychoanalytic conceptions and emphasizes therapist-patient attunement.

Integrative Specifics

Patients often approach us with relatively specific problems, such as getting anxious driving on highways, anxiety when awakening, panic attacks at work, and other interferences with daily living, the type of issues recently highlighted by Buechler (2019). Other more severe disorders are also presented, such as psychotic thinking and addictive tendencies. In all cases the patients are seeking symptomatic relief. We see these disorders through both a psychoanalytic and a behavioral lens. We consider the developmental paths that could be leading to and supporting the problems. We also discuss alternative solutions and it is the latter upon which patients tend to focus.

We know that understanding and relational support are not sufficient to change behavior, at least not in a relatively brief period, which is what is usually available. The patients want behavioral change, namely symptom alleviation, as quickly as possible. As a result, it is of considerable value to offer some direct behavioral change, which is also enhanced by understanding and a willingness to translate insight into action.

This means that we will discuss methods of anxiety reduction and possible changes in thinking and relating as ways to alleviate symptoms. We do use suggestions, but with an awareness that transference can cause patients to feel that they are being given directives, so it is important to stress that these are some possibilities rather than instructions that must be followed. A similar situation can occur with interpretation being seen as criticism rather than a possible explanation. If this occurs we discuss the patients' feelings about these issues and clarify the fact of choice for patients. Also, Eagle (2018a, 2018b) has indicated that transference interpretation and resolution are not essential to patient improvement. We are always aware that there will be resistance to replacing the old, familiar, but unsuccessful behavior with something new. A supportive relationship with the therapist emphasizes that the ego strength available to the patient is essential. Also, some patients appear to have deficits, essentially developmental lags, which will require learning new skills, particularly interpersonal, although at times, cognitive as well.

There is a significant amount of evidence to support the value of exposure in reducing anxiety. Exposure involves understanding and awareness as well as actual behavior. Suggestion is used as a way to develop possibilities such as unconscious motivation as well as other ways to behave. Our emphasis is on patients doing what works for them, but within the reality of troubling emotions such as anxiety and depression.

We believe that it can be useful for patients to also use medication because it can ease symptoms and facilitate talk therapy. However, the idea of achieving anxiety-free or depression-free existence is unrealistic. We discuss with patients different possibilities from what they are doing currently, which first involves hearing their stories so that we know about what they are doing. We support the idea of change based on evidence of the ineffectiveness of current behavior.

The idea of change is usually verbalized as acceptable but resisted in practice because while it creates hope it also brings anxiety and the latter often wins out as a determent. Medication has the appeal of anxiety reduction, but it usually does not eliminate the problem. In our experience, it can be a useful adjunct to talk therapy, but patients must understand the need for the combination.

Behavioral changes are resisted in a variety of ways. One is that the patient describes the mind as though it was an uncontrollable entity separate from the self. For example, a patient will say, "I tried to do that but my mind will not let me." This necessitates discussing the fact that the mind is part of the self, which often results in considering the idea of a split self, each part struggling for dominance with different motivations. Once a patient takes ownership of "my mind," the resistance is modified. Psychotic patients tend to limit this by creating external entities, delusions, and hallucinations, so it is necessary to develop an acceptance of the patient's creative role and then look at the motivation for the creation.

A technique that can be useful in deflecting the impact of symptoms is to accept the idea of the patient having a disorder, which is reinforced with a psychiatric diagnosis, but to have the patient see that as ego-alien, a split-off part of the self, a "not-me," while the patient also has a functioning self that is being undermined. This is different than taking ownership of a "false self," of "my mind," but it can be used temporarily as a bridge to accommodate a functioning self while it is symptomatic. Ultimately the aim will be to establish ownership of the entire self.

Distraction is also a useful method to relieve unpleasant feelings, though patients may assert that they cannot distract themselves, but with some support they usually can do this. Of course, distraction is a temporary fix, but it provides time and mental space for the patient to function on understanding the problem.

Etiology

We see symptoms as signals of more elaborate problems and suggestive of origins, although we know that they are usually at best, correlates. For example, obsessive compulsive disorders are often defenses against aggression, though not infallible clues. There is some support for the possibility of developing a developmental map of the patient's life. An intriguing question is the reasons that people differ in reaction to what appears to be the same type of developmental stressors. Also, in each individual there tends to be variable reactions. The search for the possible etiology of specific mental disorders, accepting the imprecision involved in the nomenclature, has some possible support in the concepts of ego psychology, although that was not developed primarily as a clinical exploration. As clinicians we are presented with problems in living and being asked by the patients who have them to help resolve the problems. Psychoanalysis provides a broad framework of a person, divided traditionally into id, ego, and superego, with each part having specific functions. It also indicates that the functions can conflict and that symptoms arise from the conflicts. This is basic stuff, a broad outline, but it makes the point of valuing the interacting parts of an individual and trying to understand what happens as one lives.

The ego is a major player in these conflicts regarding their resolution process which can be disruptive and maladaptive when sufficient harmony is lost. Thoughts, emotions, and behavior can and do get out of control, conflicts occur within and between people, and life becomes an emotional struggle. Although traditional analysis did not give it that much emphasis, an enduring problem is the hostility that gets generated, accompanied by attempts to mitigate it and neutralize it, but putting out one fire is side by side with another disturbance. It is no exaggeration to look at life as a continuous conflict, and as clinicians we are tasked to help people live in peace with themselves and others.

As a result, when presented with a symptom we are interested in its alleviation and we look for possible origins to find a way to help us understand the current behavior. The ego can be seen as a useful nominal term for being the mediator, namely a container of functions that can regulate behavior. One can quibble with the specifics, but the functions are essentially organizers of the personality. Bellak and Meyers (1975) presented a list that has stood the test of time enough to be reiterated by Eagle (2022). The functions are judgment, reality testing, drive regulation, object relations, thought process, adaptive regression in service of the ego, defenses, stimulus barrier, autonomous functions, and sense of mastery and competence.

These functions are of interest, but the clinical focus begins with motivations, so the underneath issues connected to the functions are the conflict between drives and subsequent compromise formations expressed in the symptoms. There is an interest in ego strength and weakness, preceded by our interest in the experiences contributing to structural functioning. Understanding begins with awareness of conflicts, as a lack of attachment, which then contributes to ego functional weakness. It is also possible that there is an inherent ego weakness that results in a deficit that is also affected by conflict, but more frequently the conflict precedes the functional limitations.

Although diagnostic categories tend to be loosely organized and there is considerable comorbidity, the categories provide some direction. In support of unearthing etiologies, but not supplying specificity, there is the idea of a "p factor" noted by Eagle that indicates high comorbidity, suggesting ego impairment in various psychopathologies. Functions noted include emotional dysregulation, deficits in response inhibition, and negative emotionality. In terms of more specificity, borderline patients have a high level of sensitivity to perceived rejection and the negative intentions of others, with the belief that others indeed intended to create such an impression. As a result, there is the possibility of perceptual distortion as a deficit. There is evidence, however, that mothers who have limited reflective capacity, namely limitations in understanding both their own and their infants' mental states, can trigger intense negative effects in the infants. The result can be a cycle of mother-child negativity based on the inability to reflect, or imperfect reflection, on the lack of use of their reflection based on the mothers' perceived needs.

What then does the therapist strive to do? Create an atmosphere of trust and safety while getting the patients' best impressions of their experienced life. Reflecting then on how that seems to be involved in relating to the self and others, and remaining open to possibilities, while ultimately integrating new perspectives that remain connected to the old, but in a less debilitating way. We used ego psychology for this discussion as an illustration of how a psychoanalytic theory can be applied, but our overall theoretical approach is pluralistic and integrative.

What then is curative? Palliative is probably a better word than curative, meaning "better than" or "good enough." From the patients' point of view, their functioning would have to be improved. From our viewpoint, we agree with the patients' appraisal and we are satisfied that we helped, that we did our part without having our own issues interfere; we were able to use our knowledge and experience to be helpful. In essence, we are told stories of lives being lived with an emphasis on difficulties in each person's life span. We listen with focused attention and considerable knowledge of what is traumatic and what could be facilitative. We offer portions of that knowledge to the storytellers once we have found ways to connect to the patient that enables them to hear us. We are often better at listening and theorizing than we are at enabling patients to listen to us and to themselves. The issue of connection is vital so we have to "tune in" and ensure the patient will "tune in" to us.

Consider this comment by Bolognini, "To tune in means to perceive the complexities inherent to the others internal states as well as our own" (Goldberg, 2022, p. 415). Taking it a step further, and using psychoanalytic language, "it is necessary for the analyst to tune in to the split-off and disassociated psychic parts, the defensive ego, and an inescapable ambivalence towards the object" (p. 415). That is one way to describe it, but it may not be so lucid, even to psychoanalysts. Nonetheless, we mention it because Goldberg (2022) suggests that within psychoanalysis it represents a push for an integrative approach, synergy between experience and interpretation.

The background for integration is coming to the foreground in a way that goes beyond integration within a method such as psychoanalysis. In an article in the *New York Times*, December 4, 2022, the work of Torrey who appears primarily interested in a biological basis for schizophrenia, a significant point is raised regarding mental health treatment. He provides evidence that closing long-term psychiatric hospitals resulted in inadequate care for severely ill patients. His suggested remedy for this is to provide these patients with treatment, despite assertions by others that it is an exaggerated need. In refutation, the wholesale discharge of mental patients from long-term care was high in the 1970s when it was viewed as a very progressive approach to the mentally ill. It turned out to be ill-advised, resulting in the closing of most long-term psychiatric hospitals and fostering an increased unstable population who were ill-equipped to take care of themselves and prone to harm others. While it is asserted that only 4% of violent acts can be attributed to mentally ill people, are violent acts in any number mentally healthy?

Granted the mental health system existing at that time had flaws, but a major asset was that it provided a community for people who would have trouble living outside of this sheltered environment. To do this it made use of all the disciplines, psychiatry, psychology, social work, counseling, and rehabilitation. While this was not the integration of treatment methods that we are advocating, namely psychoanalytic-behavioral therapy, it was more integrative than the current hospitals, many of which no longer even have a psychology department. Deinstitutionalization may have been well-intentioned, but it has been ineffective, a significant misjudgment of the capacities of the severely mentally ill to live in a less protected environment, and of the need for long-term care facilities. Today one searches in vain for public facilities that provide long-term care which has become even more of a need now than it was in the past, given the increase in addictions. Providing outpatient treatment is of value, but tends to be sporadic and short-term, thereby missing key features of the problem. Treatment for emotional disorders requires skilled providers, long-term care facilities, and therapist control of the course of therapy. Such possibilities now exist only for people who can pay for them, a fraction of those who need the help. The focus today, supported significantly by insurance companies, is on abstinence and release, despite the evidence of high recidivism. At best, the results are temporary solutions.

The policy of mandated forms of treatment is only useful if the treatment is effective, but at this time it is not that effective, so basically more treatment, mandated or voluntary, will have modest results. It is akin to jailing people with the hope of rehabilitation when the rehabilitators lack the skills to rehabilitate. This brings us to the crucial issue that effective mental health treatment requires training people to facilitate it. Current training is limited by its specific emphases, namely psychiatrists who do not do talk therapy, psychologists and social workers who cannot give medication, and a host of other helpers who are even more limited in their ability to help. The scope and complexity of mental health problems and their solutions remains unappreciated and in turn, undertreated.

In another *New York Times* article on December 7, 2022, the point is made that there is a pressing need for mental health services. A medical responder for 20 years made the following comment: "We have burned down the house of mental health in this city. . . . What New York, like so many cities around the United States, needs is sustained investment to fund mental health facilities and professionals offering long term care. This effort would indeed cost millions of dollars" (Almajera, 2022, p. 6).

Of course, cost is well recognized, and with that in mind, medical care has been turned over to insurers, a solution that rests on their willingness to provide optimal care, regardless of cost. That is a poor business model, so it is not followed. Care is instead limited by cost to the degree that insurers deem sufficiently profitable and the decisions about it are taken away from providers and their patients. The implication of using this "managed" approach is that if left to the people giving and getting the care they would provide excessive care and the result would be excessive cost. There is no evidence to support this assertion, but an assumption was made the "insurance managers" would be the most effective controllers of the quality of health services. The existing situation suggests that profit, not quality of care, is their focus. Thus, the breeding ground for recent slogans such as "Medicare for all." We have already suggested that the "right to health" bears more consideration and fiscal support than it gets, and added to that we suggest that it be managed for quality and effectiveness by people whose motivation is connected primarily to those standards. Having lived in the "COVID years" should be sufficient to make the point that whatever it costs to ensure a healthy society, those funds must be forthcoming, but that type of thinking is not being extended to mental health.

The character of mental illness involves considerable confusion and difficulty understanding what is involved and what needs to be accomplished. Mental health is not a fit for accurate prediction regarding the time needed for effective treatment or the most appropriate treatment procedures. It is both a relatively unpredictable need, but a very necessary one for a functioning society. It seems unhealthy to keep reducing payment for psychotherapy services, for example, but that is what has been happening with Medicare. That attitude drives away providers, limits potential providers, and in turn reduces the facilities available for treatment despite an expanding population of older and disabled people who need the services. This approach is costly rather than cost-saving, and it is dangerous, given the upheaval that is appearing in our society. We reiterate, the right to health belongs to all people, and our society needs to make that more of a priority.

The Nonanalytic Patient

Keeping in mind our concern with the use of psychoanalytic procedures and concepts with the "every person patient" means that we are advocating working from a position of solving problems by developing in the patient an awareness of unconscious motivation. This awareness can enable patients to alter their behavior in ways that go beyond what is likely to occur using only behavioral methods. Such an approach is likely to be met with resistance because these patients tend to have presenting symptoms that remain despite interpretations and relational interactions. The patients also need behavioral coping methods to mitigate symptoms that are usually forms of anxiety and/or depression and also tend to be reduced by medication. We use a balanced approach with all the possibilities noted being available to us and the timing and frequency of their approach based on our judgment of what is necessary to reach each patient and engage them in the treatment process. The following are examples of the type of patient that is typical of most people currently seeking treatment.

The first patient is an elderly man who has periods of severe depression as well as significant anxiety upon awakening each day. He also has numerous somatic complaints, such as stomach pain and pain in other areas of his body. All the somatic complaints have been examined by physicians and diagnosed as psychosomatic. A psychodynamic formulation indicates developmental deprivations and desperate attempts at interpersonal connections. His actions in trying to get love have been inappropriate, inducing severe guilt and self-recrimination. The role of victim, involving continual suffering and numerous brief hospitalizations, appears to be his favored way of relating, despite disavowals of desire for such a role. He has developed some insight into the dynamics of his problem and is willing to explore his tendency to resort to masochistic behavior in attempting to derive love. At times he does display better ego strength, but his symptoms get in the way of consistency. At times anxiety and physical complaints are experienced as "too much pain" and an obstacle to change. He then focuses on symptom removal rather than exploration and understanding of the symptoms that have the potential for mitigating the need for the symptoms. As a result, it has been useful to integrate both medication and behavioral methods to provide sufficient relief so that he can function to the degree that he can analyze his behavior.

Another difficult case is a woman who insists on weight reduction to the point that her overall health is at risk. She was raised by parents who valued thinness and exercise and considered themselves models for her, but they stopped short of her level of limited eating and excessive exercise. Her desire to win parental approval was excessive, resulting in a mixed message that supported rigidity, though a less excessive version that she did not incorporate. They were also forced at times to get her treatment for the actual semi-starvation. They had to switch to a message of her eating more, but their approach was viewed by her as a temporary variation as she held fast to, "slim is in, so watch it or you will get fat." The result for her is a belief that she is fat and that emotional safety requires ritualistic behavior, such as hoarding, weighing food, excessive exercise, and a preoccupation with what she eats. In addition to exercise, her limited weight is maintained by a strict diet that restricts both the type and amount of food she eats and the time that she eats.

She has had numerous hospitalizations and has been in many programs designed to normalize her weight. She "waits out" the programs, gaining enough to satisfy the program so she will be released, and then she goes back to her former approach. She views the programs as a process of "getting out" by "getting through." Before her current therapy she has had many therapists. In all cases there was a punitive element; an "eat more" logic based on protecting her health. Understanding why the disorder existed, persisted, and consideration of a more appropriate way to have sufficient self-esteem were not deemed important. The patient describes herself as a lesbian, and when she does get involved with a woman she will break her pattern to some degree, kind of buying into a different parent. As a result, it does seem useful to encourage socialization where she can have a romantic interest. The behavioral approach comes in here and it meets a type of object hunger that hopes for a loving relationship. Unfortunately, when these relationships fail, because her rate of adjustment is limited both in time and scope, she returns to the previous stance, so it is a temporary fix. While she has insight, seeing it possible that her reasons for the rigid pattern could even be revenge, that she may be so angry at her parents that she punishes herself to punish them, so far any behavior outside of her usual limits seems so unsafe that the thought of being different provokes great anxiety. At the same time, she does see herself as leading a problematic existence and she keeps trying to get comfortable with the idea of leading a more normal existence. In so doing she makes significant use of the therapist's acceptance and object constancy.

Another patient has a history of a lengthy marriage with someone who has failed at whatever he attempted. His failures infuriate her and lead to bipolar episodes. Attempts by the therapist at interpretations are usually refuted and experienced as criticism. She resists detailed expressions of emotion by acknowledging the feeling but quickly moving on. Although she is quite connected to the therapist and often credits him with being very helpful, she can get annoyed easily and indicate that she might terminate. She seems to present two selves, one that listens and uses what she is getting from the relationship, and another that ignores a more effective approach to justify her view of the interaction. She claims to understand the value of intersubjectivity, but rarely puts it into action. She will have many weeks in which she indicates that she is all right, has nothing to worry about, is accepting of her partner's very limited functioning, and then explode, at times blaming the therapist for how he is interacting with her. At these points it is useful to make a point of the value of listening in such a way that she can process what she feels at the time. It will be helpful if she can accept the possibility that she distorts what is happening out of anxiety. This is a type of slow-motion defense analysis, presented by the therapist's insistence on his presence and reiterating his intention to make observations that could be useful for her to entertain. At times, she does make use of new possibilities, but it remains difficult for her to learn productively.

Concluding Remarks

We covered a lot of ground in this chapter. We began with a discussion of intersectionality, a concept that has become prominent in developing criteria for the use of techniques to facilitate mental health. Although it can be applied in an additive manner, more frequently it is used to develop exclusionary criteria for delivering mental health services. It refers to therapeutic practices that have an apparent combination of negatives, such as a drug that reduces anxiety but also is addictive and causes weight gain. In the area of psychotherapy, in addition to effectiveness, desired qualities for funding and in turn, usage, have been brevity and cost reduction. Psychoanalytic methods have the intersectionality of being relatively long-term and as a result, costly relative to behavioral methods. The latter also often describe themselves as "evidence-based," but the evidence is suspect and based on available authenticated evidence, both psychoanalytic and behavioral methods appear effective, as will be amply discussed in chapter 6. However, psychoanalytic methods do take longer and so they do cost more, and this has led to their more limited use and apparent relevance in treatment. We countered this objection by pointing out that they each do similar things as well as different things, and that by leaving out what psychoanalysis does, a disservice is being done to patients. In addition, the behavioral approach supports the influence of managed care and the subsequent inappropriate decisions based on a model of brevity and cost reduction at the time of treatment. The realities of mental illness require treatment whenever needed for whatever duration is necessary. The ultimate cost of restricting access outweighs the temporary financial gains from brevity. Also, "evidence-based" is often a deceptively used term to promote specific therapies and to imply that others, particularly psychoanalytic, have no evidential support for effectiveness, which is not true. The reality is that it is difficult to evaluate psychotherapies and that even the existing evidence for effectiveness is not as substantial as we would like, but, in making the case for integrative psychotherapy, it seems sensible at least, to use all effective therapies, bringing psychoanalysis back into the picture.

The degree of effectiveness of all our therapeutic evidence is not actually that impressive, and improvement is handicapped by the difficulty in determining what works, as well as the competition among schools of therapy. Certainly, more research is needed as well as focusing on unification among therapies in service of doing better. At the moment we believe the complexity of mental disorders is such that an integrated approach would be more effective than privileging one approach. Also, the current managed care monopoly which puts insurers in control of the type and duration of treatment is a major obstacle to improvement. These decisions are handled more effectively by therapists and their patients, as it once was, and there is no evidence that it was especially costly. The need for third-party "management" is based on the reliance on insurance for health care, a "perk" that employers instituted instead of salary increases, which would have gone to all employees. Insurance cost to employers is based on the cost to insurance companies, which is based on usage by the employees, a variable. Limiting usage limits cost, so the government is brought on where the cost is likely to be high, namely among the poor, disabled, and elderly, so Medicaid and Medicare. We consider the idea a good use of taxpayers' money, and the idea of health insurance is relatively enshrined in the culture. The problem is the "management" which has removed patients and doctors from treatment decisions that are made by people who have an incentive to limit the use of service. Those decisions belong to the providers, and we see considerable delivery improvement if that occurs.

We believe the right to health, and in particular mental health, is already accepted by the existing government entitlements. At the same time, it is expensive, and it would be unlikely to become less so than it is under the existing approach. We do not know if it would be more expensive as a marketplace cost, namely determined between providers and recipients, but even at current levels, however, would be regulated with an emphasis on service rather than with an emphasis on profit. Particularly living in the time of COVID-19 has engendered a greater awareness of the need for psychotherapy and that needs to be accompanied by greater access to services, and that means increased funding that is appropriately unrestricted.

We also made suggestions regarding broader training for psychotherapists which is in accord with our valuing of integrated psychotherapies. Since psychoanalytic approaches have become the outlier, we urge their inclusion. We also make the point that psychoanalytic methods and theories are adaptable and useful for the type of patients currently seeking psychotherapy. We concluded by providing examples of how integrative psychotherapy can be used and illustrated how that adds to the value of the procedures.

6

Psychotherapy Research Outcomes
Possibilities and Limitations

Nothing in life is so expensive as illness and stupidity.

— Freud (1913, p. 133)

We are at a very important juncture in our discipline as we attempt to make an accurate determination of the degree to which a therapeutic intervention could have a beneficial effect on an individual, as described by research findings. Too many schools of thought are engaged in a fierce struggle for primacy as to what should constitute "best practice" in assessment and intervention to address psychological issues and what psychological model is best equipped to answer fundamental questions about these psychological processes and the development of psychological disturbances. Unfortunately, the struggle for primacy has taken a Darwinian turn where the one standing is crowned as the winner, based upon a vociferous advertisement of "empirically validated findings" that are construed as seemingly supporting their claims. The fundamental problem with the stubborn refusal to recognize the limits of such findings has been amply discussed by a few investigators (Cuijpers et al., 2019; Shedler, 2010/2017; Wampold, 2015). This is particularly problematic considering the fundamental errors in the interpretation of research findings normally used to support such claims, some of which we will discuss in this chapter. There are serious consequences of such errors, particularly the systematic erosion in capturing the complexity of human experiences and the lived experiences of our patients. In the end, our patients are the ones taken hostage and made the victims of this whole struggle for primacy.

The different schools of thought and resulting therapeutic orientations that are guiding the current discourse are themselves guided by a particular view of the nature of human experience, how we develop meaning, and, most importantly, how our mental lives can become derailed and seriously affect our emotional lives.

The central inquiry as to the best way (or "best practice") to assist our patients in addressing their psychological pain, and which is the primary reason why patients seek treatment/evaluation from professionals (Solms & Turnbull, 2002), remains in need of attention. We are joining our voices to the increasing number of scholars and professionals that have started to question the "what" and the "who" to determine "good practice" or "best practice" and its "gold standards." Considering the current state of our scientific enterprise guiding the discipline, we are unable to respond with any degree of certainty that current "evidence-based" interventions can be fairly and accurately applied across the board to all individuals, but particularly individuals from diverse communities. This is particularly the case because most of these interventions are based on using measures and instruments that were developed with individuals whose lived experiences were not necessarily commensurate with those from diverse communities.

Much has been made about the importance of finding common factors in what makes psychotherapy effective (Wampold, 2015). Although important, what is missing from this view is the appreciation of the unique ways these factors may operate in diverse communities, particularly individuals whose personal experience with others may be characterized by a history of discrimination and prejudice. Such a blanket colorblind approach implied in the search for common factors tends to obfuscate the specific qualities necessary to address the unique experience of these individuals. By what we mean, that what tends to do the most damage in our interaction with others is our failure to recognize and be sensitive to the individual's unique lived experiences, which may be characterized by multiple problematic encounters with intersectionality that may have left an indelible trauma, now anchored in their psychic structure and coloring and influencing their interactions with themselves and others; and that includes the relationship with their therapist/analyst.

McKinley (2011), in his commentary on "avoiding a collapse in thinking," sees the current state of affairs in the evidence-based paradigm as a logical outcome of an attempt to homogenize the human experience through experimental designs that require the identification of "abstract trends that become codified as normative," while at the same time dismissing or deemphasizing individual differences "by only revealing what is common across individuals" (p. 28). According to him, it is in the very nature of how the questions are structured in outcome studies that determine its outcome; they are specifically structured and geared at capturing through that lens how the phenomenon is then revealed. It is not surprising, then, that "our thinking becomes entrapped to see all clinical phenomena only in terms of means-ends relationships" (p. 29). It is also not surprising that the clinicians are then forced to give up their intellectual curiosity and engage in instrumental thinking, and thus driving them to execute "tactically-derived intervention" (p. 29), even when based on questionable findings.

On Determining Core Ingredients for Therapeutic Change

The search for identifying the core mechanism of change and the specific elements that promote such changes in psychotherapy has a long history in our field and that have resulted in the development of explanatory models from psychoanalytic, existential, interpersonal, behavioral, and cognitive behavioral-based interventions (Nevid et al., 2018/2021). These different schools of thoughts have made major contributions to our understanding of what may be involved in the development of normalcy and abnormal behaviors, which are the target of our interventions. These models also include recommendations for interventions for various psychological conditions, including recommendations for some specialized disorders (Beidel & Frueh, 2018; Luyten et al., 2017; Nevid et al., 2018/2021; Offer & Sabshin, 1984; Youngstrom et al., 2020). Under the best of circumstances, this rich development can lead to an enrichment in our understanding of the human experience where all the various elements identified as important by these different developments are seen as adding understanding to the complex nature of that experience. Instead, we find ourselves adopting "a survival of the fittest Darwinian approach" and rejecting many, if not all, the tenets of these different contributions. Fortunately, we are at a new stage in our scientific development where there is a concerted attempt at integrating what we know about the multiple factors influencing our mental and emotional state, about what works in psychotherapy, and identifying the core factors driving improvement in our patients.

On the Role of Common Factors

The work of Wampold (2015) has been often cited as providing an important framework to examine the core ingredients found to be responsible for promoting change. Based on findings from a series of meta-analyses, he identified what he calls "common factors," defined as "more than a set of therapeutic elements," and "that are common to all or most psychotherapies." Most importantly, they are assumed to be involved in collectively shaping "a theoretical model about the mechanisms of change in psychotherapy" (p. 270). Wampold's main focus in his meta-analyses is on identifying the basic pathways through which change takes place and the kinds of therapeutic interventions delivered to the patient through those pathways, regardless of theoretical orientations.

A crucial element identified by Wampold (2015) that emerged from his analysis of the empirical data is the development of "a meaningful/real (not mechanical) relationship between therapist and the patient" as a prerequisite for the mechanism of change to operate effectively; it also implies the crucial participation of the patient in the process of the therapeutic change as a "recipient." In this context, he discussed one specific model ("Contextual Model") that he found to be the most meaningfully adequate because it identifies and emphasizes specific ingredients that are found/assumed to help address "an identifiable deficit" (or a particular disorder) that is afflicting the individual. Here, the author is wittingly or unwittingly highlighting one of the major problems in understanding and assessing the accuracy of outcome data. It has to do with the importance of considering the unique quality of the "who" is involved in defining what constitutes a "deficit" or just a "problem" to be addressed. From our perspective, under the best of circumstances, it requires the professional (now functioning as gatekeeper) to be aware of and consider the individual's unique developmental trajectory related to the quality of attachments formed (Bowlby, 1988), and their history of intersectionality and multiple identities related to race, gender, and the like; it also requires for the professional to be aware of the history of trauma related to multiple and various experiences of immigration and discrimination that may be operating in the forefront or background in the individual and that may explain the intensity of the emotions related to such "deficit" or "problem" (Chapman et al., 2018; Sue, 2010; Sue et al., 2007; Tummala-Narra, 2021). Additionally, the professional's personal experiences in this regard should also be considered/examined as it may contribute to the professional's specific influence (bias) on their evaluation of "deficit" or "problem" to be addressed. Something qualitatively very different emerges in us as a function of these unique aspects of our intersectional experiences that are then at play in our therapeutic transactions.

The reality is that most of the empirical findings coming from psychoanalytic or behavioral and cognitive-behavioral studies are not always inclusive of multisectional factors and ethnic minority issues so that most of the reported findings cannot be easily and properly applied to the assessment/treatment of these populations. Thus, as we examine some of the psychotherapy studies about the specific components found to have a beneficial effect, we should remain vigilant and cautious about the application of these findings to culturally, racial, and linguistically diverse individuals until such a time they have been properly assessed with those populations (Zane et al., 2016).

Wampold (2015) discussed three major ingredients found to be most relevant and important to produce therapeutic benefits, regardless of theoretical orientations. He was referring to the extent to which the therapist was successful in establishing "a) the real relationship, b) the creation of expectations through explanation of disorder and the treatment involved, and c) the enactment of health promoting actions" (p. 270). He found, in this regard, that when these elements are meaningfully present in the therapeutic transaction, they can produce a positive therapeutic effect, even in patients with a history of disruptive attachments/relationships; it also requires an "agreement about the goals of therapy as well as the tasks" (p. 270) between the patient and the therapist, considered two crucial components in the establishing of the therapeutic alliance (Wampold, 2015). In this regard, he emphasized that the data support the view that the quality of the patient and what the patient brings to the table (poor and insecure attachment histories, etc.) is less important than the therapist's action (seen as the agent of change). He concluded that it is the therapist's contribution which is the most important; more effective therapists were able to form a strong alliance across a range of patients and that therapists who are able to develop good alliances with difficult patients may still be able to do good work with patients with histories of poor and chaotic attachments and interpersonal relationships.

This emphasis is a bit contradictory to Wampold's earlier statement, and thus it is important to decouple what is normally involved in what Wampold refers to as "establishment of the initial relationship" preceding any intervention and considered one of the crucial developments in the therapeutic transaction and the working "alliance." The process of establishing an alliance has been described by various psychoanalytic scholars as essential to secure and enhancing the benefits of psychotherapy (McWilliams, 2004; Safran, 2012; Weiner & Bornstein, 2009); it is a complex development whose specific elements are only assumed to be at play by its outcome. It is not just an issue of using pleasantries and niceties toward the patients, but rather it emerges as a function of the overall behavior of the therapists as a "genuine" person and as a professional; it is "the context" in which the therapeutic transaction takes place, and in which the patient's personal history is revealed, the history of trauma is elicited, etc. and as such, it is very difficult to measure and assess empirically. Extrapolating from findings on the role bias in human interactions (Comas-Diaz & Jacobsen, 1991; Sue et al., 2007), we can safely surmise that when the therapist's personal history with bias and racial, gender, or ethnic discrimination related to the patients are left unchecked and unexamined, it is likely to contribute negatively to the derailing of the development of this important component of therapy: From the adequate development of the transference to the proper monitoring of countertransference reactions. Although these transactions require the involvement of the patient and the therapist, it is the patient's willingness to trust and take in the therapist's intervention that becomes the most crucial and determining factor.

Establishing a working relationship relates to a very complex process that is put in place, often without mentation, and that may be experienced by those involved as intuitive and genuine connection or as disconnection and general discomfort (when not working), the nature of which may not be clear, and yet could have serious consequences for the outcome of psychotherapy intervention. Wampold (2015) does a very good job in this article describing the different and subtle set of information that patients avail themselves to determine their initial reactions to the therapist and the therapeutic transaction and whether these engender sufficient trust to be helpful. As he described it, "patients make rapid judgments about the dress of the therapist, the arrangement and decorations of the room (e.g., diplomas on the wall), and other features of the therapeutic setting . . . [of] whether they can trust their therapist" (p. 270). The concept of transference and countertransference in psychoanalysis (Morris et al., 2015; Weiner & Bornstein 2009) has provided a rich description of the complex nature of this process that is influenced not only by the patient's personal intersectionality and multiple identities history with other people, history of trauma, and concepts of self and others that emerged in the context of their early experiences; but it is also influenced by the therapist's personal experiences along those dimensions as well. It is these qualities that tend to guide these individuals' interactions with the world, including therapeutic interactions. Thus, the three pathways identified by Wampold (2015): "a) the real relationship, b) the creation of expectations through explanation of disorder and the treatment involved, and c) the enactment of health promoting actions" (p. 270) through which the contextual model of psychotherapy produces benefit, will have different requirements for the therapist and patient and will likely elicit different responses from the patient and the therapist, depending on each member of the dyad's personal history with intersectionality and discrimination. To our knowledge, these specific intersectionality issues in the patient and therapist have not been clearly and systematically examined in Wampold's analyses or in any other meta-analyses meant to identify specific beneficial elements in psychotherapy transactions or curative factors that are likely to produce good outcomes.

From our perspective and in keeping with recommendations by McWilliams (2004) and other sources, the best therapist is one who (1) harbors genuine, accepting, and nonjudgmental attitude toward a patient of color's life history of discrimination and its consequences; and (2) creates a comfortable "holding environment" (Winnicott, 1986b), where all painful feelings can find expression in ways that can be transformative. In the end, the best quality requires the therapist to own his/her personal biases and prejudicial attitudes by taking charge of his/her personal psychology and personal history, and suspend all judgments (Freud, 2013; Muran & Eubanks, 2020). The importance of assessing more carefully these characteristics in the therapist is supported by findings of early dropout rates among people of color (Gonzalez et al., 2011; Kadzin et al., 1995) due to many factors, but particularly to engendering a general sense that psychotherapy is not a welcoming process and that it requires a lot from them. Muran and Eubanks (2020) identified specific (unavoidable) elements that can cause ruptures in the therapeutic interaction, derailing its potential beneficial effect. Kadzin and associates were also able to identify multiple factors in people of color that increased the burden of participating in treatment as disproportionately distributed among minority families, with premature termination being greater for Black than for White families. A similar issue was raised in another study related to treatment initiation and retention among Black/African American and Hispanic/Latino/a individuals in individuals with posttraumatic conditions (McClendon et al., 2020).

That this is not just an academic exercise, and that real people are affected with various degrees of consequences, can be seen in many of our clinical examples. Freud's prejudicial view of the poor as not viable candidates for psychoanalytic intervention features prominently in psychoanalytic thinking that has resulted in overlooking important qualities that make it possible for even individuals suffering from poverty to benefit from self-exploration (Freud, 1913; Javier & Herron, 1992). Regarding the danger of a therapist's prejudicial stand, we are reminded of a Latino man in his mid-20s, new to psychotherapy experience, who got almost derailed from ever seeking treatment when he decided to reach out to a well-known therapist for consultation. He reported being nervous and concerned about communicating to the therapist his reasons for seeking treatment, which included wanting to know more about himself, clarifying his personal and professional goals, his general dissatisfaction about many aspects of his life, and particularly his difficulties with romantic relationships. The therapist was a middle-aged, intense-looking white woman with an office in the Upper Westside of Manhattan. She enjoyed a good reputation among her peers as a competent and bright therapist with many years of experience. The patient communicated to her that he had just joined his extended family after living away from them for most of his teenage years but that he was now planning to move out of the house again to pursue the next stage in his professional life scheduled to begin in the fall of that year.

He reported feeling quite uncomfortable and uneasy from the very beginning with the sitting arrangement at the office (very tight and close seatings), but most importantly being overtaken by a feeling that she did not appear to be that interested in his story by the way she looked (or did not look) at him, appearing somewhat distracted for the most part during the 50-minute consultation. To his mind, her general demeanor was that of someone who appeared overwhelmed with life. This general discomfort and sense of disconnect became evident and even more pronounced when hearing her assessment of his problem at the end: that his problem resided in his being too close to his mother and recommended for him to move away from under his "mother's skirt" by moving out of the house. Such a pronouncement made no sense to him as there was no explanation of how it was related to his current living situation and his immediate plans; he felt that she was giving a predetermined explanation of his problem with little to no relevance to what he communicated during the consultation. This lack of explanation left him more confused than when he started and wondered if he had made a mistake in agreeing to see a therapist from a different cultural and racial background.

This therapist violated all the basic tenets discussed by Wampold and others (2015; McWilliams, 2004) as being essential for the establishment of a proper and beneficial therapeutic transaction. She failed to work on creating a welcoming atmosphere and establishing a working alliance. There were no goal consensus and collaboration established, no attempt to adapt her explanation of this patient's problem in ways congruent with his cultural background, both of which were found to have strong relevance to therapeutic outcome (Elliott et al., 2011 cited by Wampold, 2015). It was clear to this patient that she did not attempt to show empathy and that, to his mind, she lacked understanding and genuine curiosity about him and his dilemma, and displayed a lack of interest in his psychological pain, all important characteristics described by Wampold (2015) to be strongly related to good therapy outcome. Muran and Eubanks (2020) made particular emphasis on this very issue when identifying factors contributing to therapist burnout and ruptures in the therapeutic transaction. In this context, they highlighted the effect of the therapist's difficulty managing their blind spots, the therapist's attachment style, and the presence of microaggressions as contributing to problems in the therapeutic alliance and countertransference manifestations. Judging from previous findings (Gonzales et al., 2011; Kadzin et al., 1995), that could have been the end of this patient's future involvement with therapy, as it could have contributed to augmenting this young man's feeling of disenfranchisement and alienation that many people of color and immigrants tend to feel when in an unfamiliar setting and confronted with hostile and dismissive interactions; it was experienced by him as a racially influenced overall demeanor on her part.

He later learned that this therapist was part of a "Sullivanian Group," a fringe group that created a type of commune in the Upper Westside in New York City, and that she had made the same recommendation to other patients coming to see her for consultation. Perhaps, this patient was a casualty of a seriously compromised professional with a serious case of over-identified psychotherapy orientation (a distorted version of Sullivan's interpersonal theory), used to pigeonhole patients into her preconceived view of therapeutic intervention of what would be curative for patients, regardless of the nature of the problem. It was an intervention in search of a patient. Unfortunately, similar situations are occurring in many institutions responsible for the training of future professionals where a monolithic approach to psychological disorders is maintained and where the range of treatment recommendations suggested is equally predetermined and limited, creating an intellectually rigid mindset with limited options, and hence ill-equipped to recognize and appreciate the complexity of the true nature of the problems the patient may be seeking treatment for.

A Shifting of Responsibility for Change

We referred previously to the view of the therapist as the "agent of change" in the therapeutic process emerging from empirical findings discussed by Wampold (2015); this refers to the skillful application of techniques by the therapist in the therapeutic process meant to lead to a specific outcome. The emphasis here is on the role of the techniques, but in the process, it deemphasizes and minimizes the role of the individuals to whom the technique is being applied. In essence, it is also emphasizing a shifting of the responsibility for therapeutic change from the patient to the therapist as "the catalyst of change," under the specific interventions originated and implemented by the therapist (McKinley, 2011). The focus here is on a description of "best practice" now defined as the thoughtful, timely, and properly/correctly applied actions of the therapist that is assumed to determine its outcome. Missing from this view is the adequate understanding/appreciation of the important role played by the patient whose ultimate improvement can be derailed by the work of the resistance (Morris et al., 2015; Weiner & Bornstein 2009). There is nothing more frustrating for a professional than to attempt to work with individuals who are not ready to take responsibility for changing and come to their sessions forced by an ultimatum from spouses or by order of the court, leaving the therapist exhausted in the attempts to engage a reluctant and unmotivated potential client. According to McKinley (2011), "what is at stake is the loss of subjectivity for both patient and therapist and the genuine opportunity for human contact" (p. 29). A patient's resistance to change will always win the day.

Our concern regarding the "who" and the "what" is to determine "good practice" and "its gold standards" becomes even more relevant when we are called to incorporate "culturally sensitive" approaches in our assessment and intervention. Here, the major problem resides in the responsibility of the professional to recognize and actively incorporate the importance of viewing the specific patient/client's unique personal qualities and not just as membership of a specific cultural group. There is a tendency to cluster together individuals coming from different cultural and linguistic backgrounds as a composite or amalgamation of different groups of individuals (e.g., white or Caucasian, Black, Latino, woman, man, immigrants) as a whole, with little or no consideration for "the uniqueness" of their lived experiences. The African American experience and the experience of those coming from Hispanic, Latino, Asian, South Asian, or European backgrounds are influenced by their different relationships to race, gender, socioeconomic status, religion, educational backgrounds, linguistic characteristics, or ecological and sociopolitical histories. Not all individuals with black skin are the same, as much as not all Latinos and Hispanics, and Asians and South Asians are the same. The experiences of Black Caribbean and dark skin South Asian, American Indians and Indians coming from Central and South American are fundamentally different and result in different views of the world and of the self (Clauss-Ehler et al., 2018; El-Jamil & Abi-Hashem, 2018; West, 2018). Thus, any attempt at simplification or reduction to empirically validated approaches without serious inclusion of these factors in the mix, run the risk of missing and denying the essential and unique quality of the human experience characterizing these individuals. Similar caution should also be maintained regarding white individuals without overlooking the crucial influential role of "white privilege" in our society which benefits white experience to the detriment of the rest of the society. Our greatest challenge in this regard is when we encounter white and Caucasian individuals as colleagues or patients who remain stubbornly unaware of that privilege and the harm caused to people of color. Nevertheless, we are still emphasizing here the importance of remaining faithful to our scientific tenets and recognizing that not all whites are the same regarding their relations to intersectionality. In the end, it is the recognition of the crucial importance of the principle of "suspending judgment" and allowing information about all individuals' unique characteristics and lived experiences to guide us in our assessment and intervention regardless of race, class, or position along the intersectionality dimension.

Where Are We in Our Scientific Enterprise?

The current state of affairs in the scientific community is the attempt to define and determine what factors are crucial in explaining patients' improvements as a function of what specific interventions (Muran & Eubanks, 2020). This issue has been dogging psychology from its inception, whether psychoanalytic, behavioral, or cognitive-behavioral in their approaches. It has been implied in the discussions/arguments about the determination of the theoretical orientations best fitted to explain and offer effective treatment for various emotional disturbances, with each orientation making claims based on what the proponent of each of these bands considers successful outcomes (Cuijpers et al., 2019). We can now see that some of that determination has to do with the patient's responses as well as factors related to the therapist. Such a humble realization is quite apparent in one of the last Freud's writings ("Analysis terminable and interminable"), where he conceded that a patient's improvement cannot be predicted only by the nature and quality of the methodology utilized (Freud, 1937). Some patients will not show improvement or permanent improvement and conditions in the patient are such that it makes improvements impossible, or ones that may require sporadic resumption of the treatment. Others have also made references to the necessary qualities required of the individuals involved (e.g., patients and treating professionals) as essentials to produce good outcomes in psychoanalytic and cognitive behavioral treatments (Bachrach & Leaff, 1978; Wright & Davis, 1994/2006).

Support for the view that external factors can be crucial in providing a context to understand therapeutic benefits was provided by Lambert in a 1992 meta-analysis. Findings from this analysis reported that an estimate of only 30% of the change can be attributed to common factors, with 15% to specific factors, 40% to extra-therapy factors, and 15% to a placebo effect (Lambert, 1992, as cited by Cuijpers et al., 2019). Extra therapeutic factors were also found to be responsible for about one-third of the improvement (33.3%) in another study, with nonspecific factors found to be responsible for about half (49.6%); that left only 17.1% ascribed to specific factors for the remaining sixth and smallest share of the variance (Cuijpers et al., 2019). Although we recognize that these are estimates in correlational studies and hence no statements about causal link can be made, they point to the importance of keeping in mind that the process of change in psychotherapy is too complex to lend itself to successful experimental manipulations. It is that very complexity related to the difficulty in controlling these extra therapeutic factors that are normally involved in this uniquely human enterprise, that makes a pronouncement about one orientation as being superior to others as having no scientific basis.

The serious examination of this literature provided by Cuijpers and colleagues (2019) offers an insightful revelation and guide on how the findings of these studies should be taken with a grain of salt and a good dosage of skepticism and suspiciousness because they are blatantly misleading. In the end, we are left with the conclusion that there is no clear evidence to support the best theoretically based interventions, only that psychotherapy is found to be effective across the board. Here is a summary of their meticulous and extensive review of the existing empirical literature in determining level/degree of support found for evidence-based treatment:

1. There is clear support for the view that traditional psychotherapies can indeed effectively treat most mental disorders we find in our practices.
2. It is also clearly supported that psychoanalytic, behavioral, and cognitive-behavioral interventions are found to be effective for various disorders depending upon what and how are measured. Included in the list of disorders for which these interventions are effective are conditions such as depression, anxiety disorders, posttraumatic stress disorder, obsessive compulsive disorder, psychotic disorders, eating disorders, bipolar disorder, and personality disorders.
3. What is not supported is the extent to which one therapy model is superior to others in this regard (Cuijpers et al., 2019; Wampold, 2015). The reason for that is that (a) these are primarily correlational studies that, by their very nature, are not intended to prove causal link of any kind; (b) most of the meta-analyses that are normally used in support of a particular therapy method are fraught with serious methodological flaws related to poor and too small sample size to result in sufficient power that can elicit enough confidence in the results;

(c) many of these studies suffer from high risk "researcher allegiance" problems that has been found to contaminate the determination of studies included in the meta-analyses under consideration. This relates to making decisions to include in the meta-analysis mostly studies of interest to the researchers due to their own allegiance to that specific orientation; and (d) the inclusion of "non-bona fide" rather than "bona fide" therapies, also found to be a pervasive problem in many of the studies examined.

"Bona fide" is defined by the authors (Cuijpers et al., 2019) as therapies that are "based on psychological principles . . . offered to the psychotherapy community as viable treatments (e.g., through professional books or manuals), and are delivered by trained therapists" and requiring "a judgment from expert raters" (p. 215). According to these authors, including comparison studies and meta-analyses "non-bona fide" studies, renders the findings of these studies uninterpretable or at least of questionable validity. Regarding "research allegiance," the authors considered such a condition as an example of "specific type of intellectual conflict of interest" in that "researchers with an allegiance toward one type of therapy are inclined to design or interpret the results of a comparative study in such a way that their preferred therapy is found to be superior to other therapies" (p. 215).

Although it is not clear how research allegiance works, the authors provided support from a systematic review that included 29 meta-analyses where they found only a moderate correlation ($r = 0.26$ and SMD $= 0.54$) between the outcome of the intervention and research allegiance, particularly with studies with a high bias risk. That this should be a serious issue of concern can be found in their reports of findings from some studies with controlled trials of psychotherapy for depression in adults where only 22% of the 289 studies could be rated as having a low risk of bias, with 29% (9/31) of those trials assessing treatment for generalized anxiety disorder, 10% (4/42) focusing on panic disorder, and 17% (8/48) focusing on social anxiety disorder (Cuijpers et al., 2016; Cuijpers et al. 2018). According to these authors, using these types of poor-quality trials as evidence can only lead to "overestimation of the effects of therapies" being assessed (Cuijpers et al., 2010, 2018, p. 223; Furukawa et al., 2014). The plead from these authors is for us to recognize that

> the best way to examine whether two types of therapy have comparable effects is to conduct trials in which patients are randomized to one of the two therapies and then examine whether the improvement in participants is comparable between the two therapies. (Cuijpers et al., 2019, p. 211)

The authors also examined another set of data emerging from network meta-analyses, considered superior to conventional meta-analyses because they make "optimal use of all available evidence" (p. 213). From these analyses, they identified the following thread:

- CBT was found to be significantly better than psychodynamic therapies for treating social anxiety disorders, findings that have been supported by other analyses.

• A significant difference was found between CBT and behavioral activation therapy for treating depression, but no significant difference between psychodynamic therapy and exposure and social skills training in that regard; they found "a significant difference between interpersonal psychotherapy and supportive counseling" (p. 212) also in the treatment of depression.

Finally, these authors also focused their attention on their examination of research data that looked at the level of impact of mediator/moderator factors on the level of effectiveness of specific therapeutic interventions. Although considered by the author as a good way to examine intervening variables that may account for the relationship between the treatment and its outcome, they were still left with many questions regarding the causal association assumed to have and what specific factors may have caused the change (Kadzin, 2007). Part of the reason for that is the realization that a mediator can be, in fact, just a proxy for one or more other variables, which then requires "multiple and converging lines of research to explain precisely how mechanisms of change result in better outcomes for the patient" (Cuijpers et al., 2019, p. 221). It must show "that changes in the mediator come before changes in the outcome" (p. 221), thus emphasizing its temporal relationship. Not an easy and/or practical task, with the cost alone creating the most obstacle; and then, the methodological nightmare that entails the proposed mediator and studies showing a dose-response relationship between the mediator and the outcome to be subjected to direct experimental manipulation. Additionally, it requires showing theoretical studies that present a plausible and convincing explanation of why and how the mediator resulted in changes in the patient (Cuijpers et al., 2019).

What Are We Left With?

In the end, we can only agree that the consistent findings from various sources are that psychotherapies of various orientations are effective in treating psychological disorders, although we are still not clear what are the specific factors and mechanisms involved in producing the benefits. Also that we are still unable to confirm with any degree of certainty evidence about "how a therapy works" and that little is known about the mechanism of change. It is clear that we must learn to live with the fact that psychotherapy is "a complex, multifactorial process," and that 'it is most likely that both common factors and specific factors play a part in the process that leads to recovery, most likely in complicated ways that cannot be captured by simple causal models" (Cuijpers et al., 2019, p. 226).

Uniqueness of Psychoanalytic-Focused Interventions

What also comes across from these analyses is the recognition/understanding of the specific ways different orientations operate in encouraging changes in their patients. We can appreciate in this context the important focus of cognitive behavioral therapies to change maladaptive cognitions in patients, and of behavioral therapies to change maladaptive behaviors. For some patients that may be all they can tolerate or are interested in. It does not mean that therapists should limit themselves in assuming that nothing else is involved in the development of the patient's symptomatology. Inherent in psychoanalytic interventions also include concerted efforts to help patients change maladaptive cognitions and behaviors associated with their difficulties, with a great distinction that these changes occur in the context of a strong dosage of a recognition that these manifestations are only the result of internal processes related to strong emotions (e.g., distress-anguish, anger-rage, fear-terror, shame-humiliation, and "dissmell"—disgust) (Solms & Turnbull, 2002; Tomkins, 1962, 1978). The fact that these emotions are generally not totally at the fingertip of awareness in the patient's consciousness, creates yet another important layer of treatment focus in psychoanalytic interventions. This type of intervention is based on the recognition that these cognitions and behaviors may be the result of a complex psychological organization whose origin may be related to unresolved traumatic events in the individual's life and are now utilized without mentation in the form of "personal script," and thus automatically deployed when the original emotions are directly or indirectly triggered by something in their environment (Allen & Fonagy, 2017).

A series of research that allows for this type of analysis was published in a recent publication by Luyten and colleagues (2017) who reported an extensive body of research on psychoanalytic-based assessment and interventions for children, adolescents and adults, as well as research on process and outcome studies in psychodynamic psychotherapies. Some of the findings discussed support the view that categorical approaches to understanding pathological manifestation have no basis on how emotions truly operate and are organized in reality; they endorsed instead a transdiagnostic approach to diagnostic classifications and to the assessment and treatment of psychological conditions (Luyten & Blatt, 2017; Waldinger & Schultz, 2017), an issue also endorsed by Beidel and Frueh (2018) in their extensive volume. Several research findings have pointed to the realization that it was more likely for co-occurrence and comorbidity to be more the rule than the exception in what may be affecting the patient's overall functioning (Widiger & Crego, 2018).

They reported in this regard that in findings from a clinical setting, 95% of individuals who meet criteria for lifetime major depression or dysthymia also meet criteria for current or past anxiety disorder. They concluded that such findings are guiding interventions where many current treatments are not so much treatment for transient states mental disorders of affect and anxiety but rather treatments "for core processes, such as negative affectivity, that span normal and abnormal variations as well as undergird multiple mental disorder" (Widiger & Crego, 2018, p. 6). And these authors suggest that it is important to view mental disorders "as resulting from a complex interaction of an array of interacting biological vulnerabilities and dispositions with a number of significant environmental, psychosocial events, that often exert their effects over a progressively developing period of time" (Widiger & Crego, 2018, p. 22).

With these findings, we are left with many poignant questions in terms of determining the core issues that may explain the individual's core pathological manifestation; so, questions such as, what is producing the mixed picture in someone with a mixed profile of depression and anxiety? Or, how to view someone with a schizoaffective disorder profile whether as a mood disorder or a form of schizophrenia? Similarly, how to understand whether someone diagnosed with a generalized social phobia whether to be anxiety driven or a personality disorder? Finally, the question of what may be driving a body dysmorphic disorder. Is it anxiety, eating, or somatoform conditions? (Beidel & Frueh, 2018; Widiger & Crego, 2018)

There are similar boundary problems raised by these authors when considering personality disorders, making it quite a challenge to clearly distinguish between personality disorders and other mental disorders, personality disorders and normal personality disorders, and different personality disorders (Widiger & Crego, 2018). Their conclusion is that it is not possible to make clear distinctions because "complex etiological history and individual psychopathology profile are unlikely to be well described by single diagnostic categories that attempt to make distinctions at a nonexistent discrete joint along continuous distributions" (Widiger & Crego, 2018, p. 22).

Psychoanalytic view on trauma adds to this fundamental approach of the need to shift our attention from "disorder-centered to a person-centered approach to treatment . . . or a life history perspective." The focus of psychoanalytic treatment intervention is to attempt to "map the myriad complex pathways from early childhood to later adaptive or maladaptive development" (Allen & Fonagy, 2017, 165–166). It is this specific knowledge that provides the necessary information to guide the most adequate basis for interventions for both preventing and treating disorders. Related more specifically to the role of trauma in symptom formations, Fonagy and associates' work (Fonagy & Luyten, 2009; Fonagy & Target, 1997) on mentalizing and attachment organizations provides us with a much more sophisticated understanding of how the impact of traumatic experience in one's functioning can be predicted by examining the quality of these two important components of the human experience. In this context, they see a convergence in findings from cognitive-behavioral in explaining the importance of mentalizing or the ability to attend "to mental states in self and others and interpreting behavior accordingly" and where the experience of trauma involves in part "an absence of mentalizing" (Allen & Fonagy, 2017, p. 166). In the end, regardless of the treatment orientation, the best treatment approach is the one that can successfully create "a secure attachment context conducive to mentalizing in which previously unbearable emotional state can be experienced, expressed, understood, and reflected upon—and thus rendered once again meaningful and bearable" (Allen & Fonagy, 2017, p. 166).

The importance of this work is that it provides the necessary framework to understand empirical findings that the etiological role of trauma in PTSD is complicated. It allows us to understand and appreciate that "exposure to objectively defined traumatic events is not sufficient to produce PTSD" and that "the vast majority of exposed persons do not develop PTSD" (Allen & Fonagy, 2017, p. 167; Rosen & Lilienfeld, 2008, as cited by Allen & Fonagy, 2017). We can then understand the findings that there is robust evidence for a dose-response relationship, where "the more severe the stressor, the greater the likelihood of developing PTSD," and where even "common stressors, such as family and romantic relationship problems, occupational stress, parental divorce and serious illness or death of the loved one" have been observed to produce PTSD (Gold et al., 2005 as cited by Allen & Fonagy,

2017). The importance of considering the individual's quality of attachment as it relates to the capacity to mentalize and understanding the effect of trauma can be seen in findings where children with compromised attachment experience have been found to develop problems with mentalizing. In this context, these authors reported findings of children with these types of attachment experiences demonstrating

> poorer performance on theory-of-mind tasks, disturbances in mental representations of self and parents, limited capacity to talk about mental states, difficulty understanding emotions and accurately perceiving emotional expressions, empathic failures in relation to other children's distress, and compromised emotion-regulation capacity. (Allen & Fonagy, 2017, p. 172)

Attachment processes have been found to interact with other emotion-regulatory processes, where children with a profile characterized by avoidant-attachment combined with a profile characterized by low temperamental fearfulness were predictive of conduct behaviors two years later (Burgess et al., 2003; Hill & Sharp, 2017), findings only present in boys with high psychosocial risks (Hill & Sharp, 2017).

Mentalization has been useful in the treatment of individuals suffering from borderline personality disorders, a condition with a high degree of heterogeneity in its presentation. With clarification, interpretation, and mentalizing, transference-focused psychotherapy and mentalization-focused treatment work on encouraging the capacity for reappraisal in the interpersonal perception of the self and others (Clarkin et al., 2017). This intervention is meant to address a fundamental problem for individuals with this symptomatology where fear of rejection and problems in interpersonal interactions are central. That is also meant to address their difficulty with negative emotions. Findings from various studies with borderline patients support the view that this group tends to experience more unpleasant affect and were found to be less dominant, more submissive, and more quarrelsome in their interpersonal behavior as compared with control group (Clarkin et al., 2017; Russell et al., 2007); they showed "more disagreements, confusion, hostility, emptiness, and ambivalence in their social interactions" than other personality groups (Clarkin et al., 2017, p. 356). This profile is explained by Clarkin and associates as resulting from "information-processing biases" that may be linked to "internal beliefs, assumptions, and working models of self and others," and a tendency for these individuals to selectively remember negative information (Clarkin et al., 2017, p. 356). It is these specific internal qualities that color and guide these individuals' interpersonal behavior.

Thus, a treatment intervention that addresses these fundamental issues is then likely to have a good effect on these patients. We find in this context that what makes mentalization-based treatment (MBT), transference-focused psychotherapy (TFP), dialectical behavioral therapy (DBT), schema-focused psychotherapy (SFP), cognitive behavioral treatment (CBT), and systems training for emotional predictability and problem-solving (STEPPS) particularly beneficial is that they all attempt to address some of these central and fundamental issues in borderline patients through different pathways. Again, this emphasizes that what is important is not the therapeutic orientation as also suggested by Wampold's common factors (2015), but the extent to which they address the core psychological deficits causing the problem for the patient.

Crisis in the Academy

We are truly at a critical juncture in the field of mental health. Many training institutions are now requiring those still in training to become specialists based on a limited view of the human experience, without the necessary general foundation about the complex nature of the human experience that we, as therapists, are called to address. This issue is made even more urgent and alarming by the fact that many graduate programs are administered/managed by individuals with high (blind) adherence to a specific theoretical orientation and where the view of an "evidence-based approach" is stilted toward empirical findings mainly based on the dubious studies discussed earlier in this chapter. This is particularly problematic in the absence of meaningful exposure to other literature emerging from different perspectives that also offer an empirically validated approach while also maintaining focus on the complexity of what the patients are bringing to the table (such as the work of Peter Fonagy, Michael Solms, Sidney Blatt Chris Moran and Catherine Eubanks, and Jeremy Safran); such restrictions deprive students in training at this level from important perspectives and in the process reducing the complexity of human experience primarily into researchable/manageable chunks that can be processed and treated within their limited theoretical range. In the end, university programs are becoming more like "specialized training institutes" which is usually the purview of postdoctoral specialization training programs; the added danger is that it may result in reducing the scope of inquiry and thus likely resulting in missing the larger picture of what may be crucially at play with the patients coming to treatment, as amply discussed by Allen and Fonagy (2017) and Clarkin et al. (2017). This is the issue raised by McKinley (2011) discussed earlier, with his concern that it may result in the training of future professionals to engage primarily in instrumental thinking, and only executing "tactically-derived intervention" (p. 29).

Concluding Thoughts: In Search of Intellectual Humility

The idea that there is more commonality than differences among the various psychotherapy schools has been highly endorsed by the work of Wampold (2015) and associates (1997, 2002) but also challenged by others. Some psychotherapy schools maintain that it is their unique conceptualization and intervention that is producing the necessary outcome and is beneficial to their patient. Others maintain that only an empirically (reductionistically) validated approach should be considered in keeping with psychology as a scientific enterprise. However this debate is framed, the current state of affairs, including findings from empirical studies, endorse the view that the only conclusion that we can confirm is the benefit of psychotherapy in making a difference in the lives of many people. What is not clear is 'how' and '*what*' are the specific mechanisms producing these changes that are attributing to the psychotherapy process itself and, at times, to the therapist's specific intervention.

The fact that current empirical findings only point to a correlation, or a reflection of a therapeutic effect, does not allow us to speak about any causal relationship between these factors to clearly explain how the improvement occurs. Part of the reason is that psychotherapy is a complex process whose work is not limited to what is happening in offices, but that extraneous factors are always at play that cannot be subjected totally to empirical manipulation. Many studies of psychotherapy normally included in these analyses suffer from a considerable risk of bias, low statistical power, publication bias, and researcher allegiance (Cuijpers et al., 2019), which render their findings questionable at best and misleading at worst, call for us to remain humble concerning what we know.

There are a few elements related to the role of the working alliance that continue to emerge as a strong factor in producing good therapeutic effect even in very empirically sophisticated studies (Zilcha-Mano, 2017, as cited by Cuijpers et al., 2019) such findings point to the importance of looking at specific patient's characteristics in this regard. As discussed earlier, the "trait-like" component of alliance (with which the patient comes into the therapy), or the "state-like" component of alliance (that changes as a result of therapy), were found to play a different role during the therapeutic process. A good "trait-like alliance" was found to be "a prerequisite to engaging in therapy and making it effective," while the "state-like" changes in the alliance during treatment were found to predict the subsequent outcome; it suggests that "it is the 'state-trait' that might be responsible for making 'the alliance therapeutic in itself'" (Cuijpers et al., 2019, p. 223). However, because other unmeasured variables factors may be driving the change, we are still advised to be cautious about such a claim.

Finally, the fact that psychotherapies are beneficial, although the mechanism of change remains unknown, speaks about the complexity and yet simplicity of the therapeutic endeavor. Simplicity because one intervention may trigger/cascade into other aspects of their lives, also influenced by unknown and seemingly extraneous factors that in combination with the focus of the intervention end up improving the patient's overall functioning. So, how do we know what or who was involved in producing, encouraging, or making therapeutic changes possible? That is one of those questions that force us to be humbled. All we know is that by offering an opportunity (by creating the necessary environment) for patients to engage meaningfully in making sense of the nature of their difficulties and what is contributing to their psychological pain; that by guiding the patient in the development of a cohesive narrative about the nature of their difficulties and pointing to potential solutions, we are in more solid ground to suggest that we, as therapist, may have contributed (not determined) to opening the possibility for healing where other external factors also became available to these individuals in their determination to get to a better place.

Language and Its Vicissitude in Bilingual Treatments

This chapter addresses the central and organizing role of affects in a bilingual context, the expression and processing of which can become derailed when the therapeutic process is dismissive of the unique and complex linguistic paths through which affects find expressions in individuals with multiple linguistic pathways. The chapter is guided by the understanding that linguistic processing and expressions of experiences are guided by the very same psychological principles affecting all human experiences. That means that our relationship to language and its expression will also be guided by the same evolutionary principles always at play to ensure the protection of the organism physically and psychologically. It is at play in the various and unique linguistic expressions used by our linguistically diverse patients to communicate their psychological concerns when describing painful aspects of their inner life. We will provide clinical examples in this regard, with emphasis on describing the challenges to the integrity of the therapeutic work possible when the processing of the clinical material related to diverse cultural and linguistic identities is not properly considered in the therapeutic intervention. We argue that the greatest challenge in this regard resides in our tendency to maintain an ethnocentric perspective in dealing with the world. We also argue that failure to create the necessary condition for mentalization to take place in the therapeutic process for this population will also compromise the expression of the richness of their inner life encoded in their linguistic expressions. That requires us to allow the clinical material to emerge freely without a premature interpretation of its content.

A Case of Intersectional Trauma:
A Search for Meaning

In previous chapters we discussed several thorny theoretical and empirical issues related to the importance of widening the scope of our inquiry to allow for a more comprehensive understanding of the multiple factors that may be involved in making a difference in the lives of those engaged in psychological treatment. In that context, we highlighted specific and nonspecific factors that have been found to make changes possible in those engaged in psychological treatment (see Chapter 6) (Cuijpers et al., 2019; Wampold, 2015), regardless of the therapeutic orientations utilized. We examined, in this regard, issues related to the need to integrate different theoretical perspectives to guide our interventions in ways that are consistent with the psychological needs of our patients' unique intersectionality and multiple identities. One of these multiple identities has to do with the role of language in normal and psychopathological development, particularly relevant for individuals who have multiple linguistic registers to organize, communicate, and negotiate with their environments.

We recognize that language plays an important role in the development of the cognitive process as amply described by several scholars from neurolinguistics, psycholinguistics, sociolinguistics, and educational psychologists (Bialystok, 2001; Bialystok & Cummins, 2000; Luria, 1973, 1981; Luria & Yudovich, 1968; Piaget, 1995). We also recognize that language is intimately involved in the organization of the individual's emotional life that becomes intricately encoded in linguistic expressions. Finally, because of this close involvement of language and emotional development, we recognize that language function is also guided by the same biologically based mechanism that guides the individual's response to his/her environment; the same internal mechanism and rules that secure the survival of the organism biologically/ psychologically that was described by Tomkins (1962, 1978) in his voluminous volumes on affect development, Solms and Turnbull (2002) on the brain and the inner world, Freud (1973) and Sullivan (1953) on defense operations of the inner life and others from psychoanalytic perspectives, and also summarized recently by Javier and Owen (2020). That means that language expression can also serve a defensive function and be used as part of a maneuvering mechanism to defend against getting too close to difficult affective material, an issue that becomes particularly relevant when working with individuals who have multiple linguistic registers to organize and communicate traumatic contents affecting their general functioning. We have addressed these very issues in previous publications (Javier, 1996, 2015; Javier & Owen, 2020), and we encourage those interested in additional information on that topic to review those publications. Our interest in referring to this material here is to offer a context to facilitate a better understanding of the clinical material presented next. In these examples, we don't only witness the defensive usage of language, but the rich and demanding cultural contexts under which these patients operate, which then forces the clinician to become more flexible in the processing of the information and in the utilization of possible therapeutic interventions.

The Case Synopsis of Ms. G

Let's consider the case of a young woman of Latin American and Caribbean origin (whom we will call Ms. G in treatment with one of the authors and thus the pronoun "I" is used when appropriate); she presented with an urgent request for professional intervention for her mother from whom she had been estranged for most of her early history. There was a mixture of emotional distancing in the presentation of her mother's dilemma as if speaking about someone toward whom she did not have much emotional investment in; and yet, at the same time, showing a great deal of concern and despair for her mother's condition, as if it was an intractable illness. She reported that she had received a recommendation from a colleague and expressed relief that she finally found someone to take "care of my mother." Reportedly, this was not the first attempt to get her mother in treatment who either initially had not agreed to or, if she did, actively sabotaged any consultation with anyone by refusing to attend the session at the last minute. Not surprisingly, we will soon find out that this time it met with the same fate as before, adding to Ms. G's feeling of hopelessness and helplessness. It was a predictable behavior related to her mother's script characterized by a series of unstable and abusive relations with men with questionable histories. She was described as having unstable work history in the entertainment industry where her attractive body and singing voice provided her with an opportunity to survive but also attracted unsavory characters. In that context, she developed a personal script colored by having spent all her life trying to avoid any situation where strong emotions are involved and escaping into alcohol and other substances in search of emotional numbness.

Her mother agreed to attend the consultation only after Ms. G threatened to start the process of removing her still-underage half sister legally from her care now that she (Ms. G) was in a financial position to do so. Ms. G also reported having a brother who was not in the picture as he dropped out of any relationship with the family soon after reaching emancipation age, and she now has no connection with him. Ms. G presented herself as someone who was now heading a business in the garment industry that was earning her good dividends and thus allowing her a more comfortable life. Ms. G also reported that she sought the services of a bilingual/bicultural therapist because she needed someone for her mother who spoke Spanish to facilitate communication about a complicated life experience that her mother has not made sense of or spoken about with anyone.

But there was also a sense in the intensity of the presentation that it was a much more personal motivation at play for Ms. G. There was a sense that she had firsthand knowledge of what was in store for her sister and how psychologically compromised her mother was. There was a sense that, although Ms. G seems to be primarily driven by a strong desire to protect this sister, she was trying to address an old issue having to do with her complicated relationship with a mother who abandoned her at a vulnerable age (seven years old), and leaving her alone to deal with her confusion and frustration, her intense feelings of anger toward her and those around her, her strong resentment, and a profound disappointment. There was a sense of a profound void and despair that she was trying to address in the process, her need to understand her feeling of abandonment, and the reason for her mother to just pick up and go, leaving her behind. But at this point, what was prevailing and most prominent in her conscious mind was her feeling sorry for her mother, a state that allowed her to be responsive to her (mother's) demand for financial and emotional care from her, although she was unable to provide the same for Ms. G while growing up when she needed it and longed for it the most.

There was a tremendous sadness in her eyes when the therapist finally met with Ms. G and a strong sense of desperation in her use of the language, her tone, and her hand gestures; it felt as if she was reaching for her last straw before hopelessness set in. What was interesting was that she decided to speak English during this initial encounter and the earlier meetings with the therapist, although Spanish was her first and primary language, while also seeking a Spanish-speaking professional for her mother; perhaps, her need to create some emotional distance. There was a sense that Ms. G was much more overwhelmed with intense and complicated feelings than what she portrayed by her outward presentation.

Taking refuge in a second language narrative may be providing sufficient emotional distancing for Ms. G to make it possible to maintain her new identity, while also protecting her from the emotional turmoil associated with her earlier abandonment experience and feelings associated with the resulting *forced identity*. We call it "forced identity" because it is not something that was initially self-generated by the patient but forced by the circumstances and assisted by the acquisition of a different linguistic register (English) to organize and process her subsequent experience once she arrived in the United States. Buxbaum (1949) and Greenson (1950) pointed to that very process in their early writings, and most recently by Javier (1995, 2007), Javier & Lamela (2020), and Perez-Foster (1996). A second language could provide an opportunity for emotional distancing and establishing of a personal identity characterized by defensive maneuvering and a false façade as someone well-put-together but with a precarious inner life. Winnicott's (1974) concept of "false self" is relevant here as it provides a good description of the extent to which an individual would go to protect itself from psychological disintegration.

Under the development of that new persona, Ms. G appeared well-put-together, with a clear goal and determination in her presentation. She was a young woman in her late 40s and casually but stylishly dressed during her meetings with the therapist on a hot summer evening; that included her jewelry (earrings with precious stones and diamond ring), matching purse, long beige dress that allowed her to sit comfortably (covering her legs), and softly applied makeup. She tended to lean forward and look at the therapist intensely while speaking as if making sure to express the seriousness of her plight. There was also a slightly seductive tone in her presentation of an innocent little girl seeking the attention or care of an adult considered to have paternalistic qualities.

Her mother, on the other hand, came to the consultation in a black dress with a large red flowers pattern, black shoes, a purse (which she kept pressed against her chest for the whole consultation), gory-looking jewelry, heavily applied makeup around her eyes, and deep red color lipstick. In all, giving the appearance of someone who had appreciated dressing elegantly before but who now was trying hard to force a good appearance, as if getting ready for a performance. When speaking, the mother tended to avoid looking at the therapist and instead allowed her gaze to roam around the room aimlessly without attempting to pause at any specific item in the office.

Multigenerational Trauma

It was clear from the very beginning that Ms. G's request was for a multigenerational trauma intervention that included her mother, her sister, and her absent brother, the effect of which she was so desperately attempting, but unsuccessfully, to avoid being affected by it. This is not an unusual request, as a similar request was made by a Dominican-born young man who, after many years of financial struggle, established a lucrative business in the supermarket industry along with his other brothers. Coming from a large family of sixteen brothers and sisters, he too requested to have family meetings with the whole extended family once he was in treatment for several years and finally got his emotional and romantic life on track. He even referred his younger brother for treatment a few years after termination of his own treatment. This brother was struggling with similar issues with his wife and children and suffering from debilitating symptoms of agoraphobia and fear of flying.

We see this sense of personal responsibility for the welfare of the whole family in many Hispanic families (Javier & Lamela, 2020; Javier & Yussef, 1998; Paniagua & Yamada, 2013), as instilled by cultural expectations that those in better financial situations should assist those in the family with needs. These culturally anchored expectations become an essential component of these individuals' self-definition and a personal script that guides their behavior with themselves and others (Dana, 1993). It is that profound sense of family responsibility that leads many immigrant families in the United States and other countries also to continue to send money (*remesas, remeses,* or remittances) to support their families still in the countries of origin, even if depriving themselves in the process of important financial resources for their own survival in the new country. To view that behavior simply as guided primarily by guilt and the inability to separate and develop one's own autonomy is reducing a complicated culturally motivational matrix that may be guiding such behavior to a simple expression of psychopathology.

The request to treat other family members may present a tremendous challenge for a professional, particularly if trained primarily in individual treatment, or even when also trained in other modalities. We may have been strongly advised to avoid mixing treatment modalities in our training for a multitude of reasons: it may create a conflict of interests or create a messy clinical situation related to possible treatment collusion, loss of boundaries, loss of objectivity, etc. It will require the professional to establish clear parameters ahead of time where individual privacies are zealously maintained, and members of the groups are given opportunities to talk and listen to one another about their experiences under the close guidance and therapeutic eyes of the professional. It requires close adherence to remaining objectively anchored as a neutral and genuinely open-minded participant in the transaction (with the suspension of all judgment). When this process is possible, it does allow the professional a more direct opportunity to witness what may be creating the current problem for the patient and a more direct and unique understanding of various ways transgenerational trauma dynamics related to the relationships with different generations (patient's mother and grandmother, etc.) were created and now likely affecting the patient's current functioning.

The development of such an intense feeling of responsibility by Ms. G toward her mother's and sister's well-being was particularly intriguing since she did not grow up with them after her midteens. According to the history provided by Ms. G, she reunited with her mother only recently when her mother immigrated to the United States with the patient's sister, while running away from an abusive family relationship and an undefined threat to her life. Her brother decided to stay in the country of origin, while still disengaging from the rest of the family. When inquiring as to what was creating the urgency for a consultation at this time considering her mother's chronic history of emotional instability and abusiveness, it became clear that in Ms. G's mind "the situation with my mother have reached a boiling point." As Ms. G described the current situation, she indicated that her mother was now behaving obsessively with her sister by attempting to control all her ins and outs, and being extremely and intensely overprotective, a far cry from her previous neglectful and self-centered attitude while in the country of origin. Ms. G reported to be very concerned about her sister who recently had to run away from home. She reported that her mother was harassing this sister for being out too late, a behavior that her mother referred to as "not the behavior of a respectful young woman" and her stated concern of what others will think of her as a mother.

Vicissitudes of a Traumatic Life

Ms. G reported little interaction with her mother while growing up in Panama. Her mother frequently disappeared, leaving the patient to the care of her maternal grandmother and other extended family members who would take turns to provide minimally for her until her early teens. She reported her experience during that time of being assigned to housecleaning and the most demanding house chores as if she became identified as *la sirvienta* or forced servitude for the whole family. The patient reported that she decided to uproot herself from that chaos that had also resulted in her being sexually abused when still a little girl by people known to her grandmother, who was also described as having a checkered history. Feeling alone and unprotected, she decided to leave the whole family in Panama to come to the United States while still a minor, "as an act of desperation," to save her soul. It was that total disregard for her well-being by her mother and extended family, and her constant reminder by the grandmother of her being seen as a burden to the family, that prompted the patient to find an escape. It was clear by her description that her mother's franticness and unstable emotional outbursts and heavy substance usage even in her infrequent visits, was now becoming unbearable and emotionally draining and debilitating for the patient. We can see here also how this patient felt compelled to take a drastic step by abruptly uprooting herself from the family, refusing all contact in much the same way her younger sister was now engaged in attempting to do and their mother had done many times before, by dropping out of the family and engaging in a life of cabaret instead, in their desperate attempts to leave behind a chaotic and toxic family environment.

Despite that history, she reported great concern for her mother and was now prepared to assist her as a final attempt "to help her get better." She described her mother with some modicum of compassion as someone who had a very difficult life, who has been traumatized and abused while in the country of origin, and who desperately needs to talk to someone professionally about her experience, to help her "get it out of her." Part of that complicated experience included her mother not having an opportunity to speak about her own sexually and physically abused history by close family members while still a minor and her decision to escape her home while still a young woman in a desperate attempt to save herself.

It was clear from her presentation that she was viewing her mother as a tragic consequence of the same family environment she (patient) was running from, and that the toxic nature of that environment deprived her of having any relationship with her mother, rendering her an orphan of love. It was also clear that she was now engaged in a desperate attempt to rescue and repair that mother with the hope that once she was more psychologically stable it would allow her to resume her role as the mother that Ms. G so desperately was longing for (Winnicott, 1965). In her mind, the sense of franticness in her mother's multiple failed relationships following her decision to leave home and the desperate ways the mother made decisions to become involved in these multiple relationships that resulted in different fathers to her, her brother, and her younger sister, was just the tragic consequence of having been exposed to her toxic family environment.

In presenting her plea for her mother's treatment, Ms. G also made it clear that she was ok and that she was already in treatment with a female psychologist in the city whom she saw when needed. She also reported that she was comfortable with that arrangement and that she communicated in English with this therapist. She described her treatment as basically discussing practical issues about her life and that most of the sessions were not regularly scheduled and only focused on giving her specific advice that she found helpful. She saw it as a business transaction. It was as if she did not expect much from this female therapist, just as she did not expect much from her own mother. This arrangement was found most acceptable because she was able to control the contact and limited it to only getting some guidance when she needed it.

Following the consultation and the mother's refusal to return for treatment after the first and only session, Ms. G reported that she realized how much she had inside her and wanted an opportunity now to discuss her concerns with the therapist initially requested for her mother. She looked surprised when it was recommended that she needed to have that conversation with her previous therapist before switching treatment with me, considering the long period she has been in treatment with that therapist. This is an important intervention for someone whose family history includes proneness to just leave a situation found intolerable. The possibility for this type of reenactment in treatment was seen as quite likely, particularly when the material emerging in her treatment becomes too intense. We have seen in patients with this kind of trauma history a tendency to break the treatment when facing strong emotions and then return a few weeks or months later to resume. We may consider such a break "an act of enactment with a purpose" if the patient resumes the treatment. When such an enactment does not allow the patient to resume, it suggests that it was too painful and disorganizing for that patient and hence the need to tread gingerly should the patient return at a much later point, due to the level of fragility demonstrated by the escape.

I Have Feelings Too: Navigating Her Emotions in Two Languages

For the first meeting Ms. G selected English to communicate, something that she did relatively well, but found herself switching to her primary language in her treatment when unable to find a good way to proceed in English; this usually happened while relating some of her mother's "crazy behaviors." Nevertheless, there was a sense that it was very important for her to speak English despite her struggle and even when she had the option to speak in both languages.

Her first order of business was her request for assistance in handling her mother and guidance for her sister, in the context of which the therapist began to get a better sense of the nature of her difficulties dealing with her mother; it was related to her deeply engrained sense of obligation as her older daughter, despite the history of neglect and her strong feeling of ambivalence. She reported feeling profound guilt about her frequent need to avoid her mother and for zealously trying to protect her personal space from being contaminated or messed up by her mother and her craziness. She also reported her frequent use of alcohol "*para relajarme*" (to relax) at the end of the day, which she would do as she listened to her favorite music in Spanish, feeling quite nostalgic at the end. While listening to the music, she reported that she would eventually join in the singing, which inevitably included reliving memories of her childhood and finding herself sobbing with tears of longing for the recognition and care that she never had; it would then turn into anger when remembering the many rejections and the feeling of not belonging that she endured.

Ms. G described her early experience in this country as extremely difficult as she was dealing with a strong feeling of loneliness, limited knowledge of English, no family she felt she could lean on, but armored with a determination to make it work, where failure was not an option. That meant her working long hours in various menial jobs that allowed her to survive financially and always relying on her constant companion (marijuana) "to calm my nerve." With her clear determination and getting progressively better command of the language, she landed a job in the corporate world; in that world she eventually met someone with whom she would allow herself to become romantically involved and with whom she eventually started a successful business in the garment industry. She initially described this relationship as a supportive one, and him as someone who was not demanding and was "family oriented." She also reported English as the only language of communication between them because of his limited knowledge of other languages. She eventually would report a feeling of emptiness and unsettledness, often unable to reconcile her sleep and relying on the use of marijuana or a few glasses of wine regularly "to calm my nerves down" and be able to sleep.

Her main struggle in this relationship, as it was with previous relationships with other white men of European background, was her feeling that she needed to work and try harder, struggling with a feeling of not belonging, or relying on her natural beauty as a woman to keep him interested in her (here we see a parallel to her mother's own journey). She also reported a feeling of resentment in his treatment of her. This was related to her experience of being excluded by him from important business decisions and that she considered a lack of respect on his part for her intellect and her capability as a businesswoman. She reported having difficulty sleeping and being constantly worried about finances and having stable living conditions. What emerged from the exploration of her difficulty sleeping was her fear that once she closed her eyes, the whole emotional mess and images of her past would take over her mind and show in her dreams. She reported frequent dreams in Spanish where she felt alone to face dangerous assaults from faceless man figures or animals that were able to attack her. In many of these dreams she was able to prevail and be ok. Here is an example of these dreams now translated:

> I found myself at the family finca (hacienda) where there were all kinds of animals around, but I wanted to prepare a seafood meal for which I was now carrying all the ingredients to the kitchen in bags. I placed the bags on the kitchen counter and as I was taking out all what was in the bag, the first thing that I brought out was a snake, 'a green and beautiful snake'. Surprised, I attempted to stretch it and place it on the kitchen counter, but the snake curled and wrapped itself around my fingers and eventually bit me. Although initially concerned that it was poisonous, I realized that I was ok. I then tried once again to stretch the snake on the counter and again the snake wrapped itself around my hands and fingers and bit me. I now noticed that I had two-hole marks in one of my fingers and some blood showing on that finger. I started talking to the snake telling her to stop biting me and it bit me again. I then stretched out the snake but that now seemed dead and not moving when I placed it on the kitchen counter. It stayed there.

This dream was presented at the very end of the session with an announcement that there was a second dream following the previous one, which the patient communicated in the following session.

> In that dream, I was caring for an elderly woman whom I was carrying on my shoulder and who was in urgent need to go to the bathroom when I suddenly felt that the elderly woman had shit on my shoulder, and now I was carrying feces on my shoulder.

These dreams were communicated in both languages although they took place in a Spanish context and related to Spanish themes. They are full of symbolism regarding her complicated feelings with people around her, which required a sensitive approach from the therapist in eliciting her associations as to possible meanings in her life. For that, a combination of Spanish and English was used in the intervention, allowing the patient to discuss the content of her dream in the linguistic mode she felt most comfortable. It was clear that she was disturbed by her dreams by the fact that she waited until the end of the session to communicate the first one, so as not to have to delve too much into the possible meaning; and by her need to turn the theme of the second dream into something positive when asked for her association to the dream. She reported, in this regard, that she woke up excited about dreaming about feces on her shoulder because "to dream about feces meant that something good was coming my way." Regarding the first dream, it seems a reflection of the dangerousness she has experienced in critical areas of her life related to even basic needs (food); it also revealed her murderous (but detached from her consciousness) feelings against those that cause her pain and harm, which although she was initially afraid of great harm (being poisoned) from them, she realized that she was ultimately ok, and that she has escaped serious harm. In the end, she ended up killing the snake, although in ways suggesting her refusal to engage in clear reprisal against the snake attack on her, and the denial of her murderous feelings residing in her. Instead, she rendered the snake motionless with love and tenderness, and unable to harm her, reminiscing of some of the possible reasons why she was seeking treatment for her mother.

There are some important considerations in determining what linguistic mode to use in entering an examination of inner experience with different degrees of affective impact. Due to this patient's history and her multiple identities associated with her languages, we suspect that the most disturbing experience in her life occurred in a Spanish context and likely to be more closely organized in Spanish; we also suspect that speaking about these dreams in English provided her with a welcome refuge to the potential fear of fragmentation associated with the intensity of her feelings of rejection and abandonment, while at the same time, allowing her to at least discuss and come to terms with some of the components of these experiences. In the end, only when the patient can return to the original location of these disturbing feelings (Spanish), we begin to consider the possibility of integration of the different aspects of herself associated with her multiple identities.

The decision to use one or another language of a patient to explore or address central issues of the patient's life characterized by intense emotions (like when dealing with traumatic events) is a very delicate enterprise that should consider the patient's normal defensive maneuvers to deal with difficult emotions. Although there are individuals who insist on communicating in a second language as a component of their regular tendency to use intellectualization to avoid access to their emotions, others may do so just to get some respite from the overwhelming impact of strong emotions that could render them cognitively and emotionally disorganized. Ms. G seems to belong to this latter group. With patients who are prone to suppression of affect like Ms. G, the second language could be used as a bridge to allow discussion of suppressed material likely to result in the presence of disorganizing effects. Patients with a tendency toward intellectualization to negotiate disturbing affects may find additional refuge in a second language to provide additional opportunities to gain distance from this important material; in that case, patients should be encouraged to speak in the first language when ready for a full sense of the extent of these emotions. Patients who are prone to become too disorganized with emotions may use the second language to communicate the content of these emotions, a maneuvering that should be respected. However, without engaging in the language of the primary emotions, we cannot determine the extent to which these patients can accomplish full integration of their multiple identities and reach emotional stability.

In Search of Her Father

When the patient allowed herself to speak about her different history of traumatic events in Spanish, there was a palpable emotional intensity in the room, accompanied by frequent impregnated and paralyzing silence, and finally uncontrollable tears; during those times, the patient sobbed as if the tears were emerging from the deepest and recondite part of her tortured soul. Such a revelation in the treatment was preceded by a question in Spanish asking "*Y qué emociones estás sintiendo en lo que me estás contando?*" (What emotions are you feeling in what you are telling me?) She looked initially stunned while providing the details of her painful past, as if in touch with raw emotions, the enormity of which was paralyzing her. She reported being surprised about the intensity of her emotions when she found herself with tears in her eyes on several occasions; she was ultimately relieved and thankful about these sessions, adding that "I guess I have feelings too."

These moments were followed by a few days of sustained sadness, difficulty sleeping, an increase in alcohol and substance usage, and a need to be alone. There were several of these moments before she decided that it was time to find out more about her father. Her memory or lack of memory of her father became progressively more centered when a family member from her father's side reached out to speak with her. It was also guided by her vague awareness of a very early memory of her father that emerged in a dream she recently had following a session where her relationship with her father or lack thereof was the focus. It seems like something was unlocked from her memory as she engaged in her primary and early language where the stubborn power of these early memories was lodged and through which all relationships with the world were ultimately filtered. We can now see that her decision to seek treatment with a male therapist with some paternalistic qualities was part of that search for a father figure. We can also see how her decision to marry an older and more financially settled man may have been influenced by this same dynamic.

On Relying on a Second Language to Forge a New Identity

We have described in previous writings how language can serve several functions in the cognitive and emotional life of the individual (Javier, 2007). Being that we have amply discussed this process elsewhere, we will only describe here briefly what may be going on with Ms. G. When listening to her story, I became concerned about the precariousness of her internal presentation, although her outer persona seems as one in complete charge of her emotional state. She was running a reportedly successful business, was on the verge of establishing a home in the suburbia, was engaged in a stable relationship with a person from a different cultural and linguistic background, and with whom English was her preferred language of communication. It looks as if she succeeded in creating/establishing the ideal life for herself, protected from the chaos that produced so much pain for her in the past. But her mother's presence was a reminder of what she was so desperately attempting to distance herself from and was a continuing threat to her ideal creation. She felt the desperate need to rescue her sister because she saw too much of herself in her sister and leaving her at her mother's mercy was as if she was reenacting her own abandonment, but now taking her mother's role. Tortured by her intense disdain (contempt) for her mother but also her keen awareness of the duty of a good daughter expected by her cultural values, she came to a compromise similar to the one used by her mother when she left Ms. G to the care of her grandmother and her mother's extended family. That was done because, in her mother's mind, she saw that her family was more financially able to care for Ms. G while she (her mother) tried her luck elsewhere. This time, Ms. G is using the financial security from her current relationship to keep her mother at bay, from disrupting her current situation. Considering her current situation, it does not look like her attempts are working well for her; even her linguistic maneuvering was not protecting her from her emotions in much the same way that smoking marijuana every day "to calm my nerve" was not providing much in the way of lasting relief, but only as a temporary refuge to her tumultuous emotions. She was finding herself in what she referred to as "*a callejón sin salida*" (a blind alley), trapped in the same predicament.

We can explain Ms. G's, her sister's, and her mother's conditions as driven by a series of unarticulated experiences of trauma that have made their lives strongly intertwined with one another. There is a history of physical and sexual abuse and neglect, as victims/witnesses of domestic violence that are now part of what Ms. G is so desperately attempting to eradicate from her past. Such a condition was described by Christine Courtois as 'complex trauma' or trauma compounded by other traumas (Courtois & Ford, 2009) that can have devastating consequences, particularly when dealing with other stressful events. It seems that Ms. G is engaged in a series of coping strategies that have made her life somewhat more tolerable for a while. Her decision to immigrate and her use of marijuana and language switching could be construed as her desperate attempt to negotiate the overwhelming impact of the ever-increasing presence of her intolerable affects.

The use of language to maneuver uncomfortable affects has been amply described by several authors over the years (Buxbaum, 1949; Foster, 1996; Javier, 2007; Marcos, 1976). That includes the use of language for distancing, as a container, and to soften the effect of negative emotions, while allowing opportunities to work through otherwise too disorganizing affect-filled materials. Language can ultimately be viewed as providing a holding environment to patients prone to the use of splitting or repression of affect to allow the exploratory work to proceed in ways that give these patients progressively more access to the content of the material that is creating the disorganizing effect in their lives.

Part of the reason for looking at Ms. G's condition through the trauma lens is the recognition that traumatic experiences reverberate in an individual's life, leaving an indelible mark in one's psychic structure that becomes a reference point to other interpersonal activities (Courtois & Ford, 2009). According to Russell (1998), trauma causes injury (physically and psychologically) that under more severe and persistent abusive conditions can render the individual helpless and hopeless and cripple one's ability to negotiate the traumatic events and their consequences. For Russell, what causes the pain is not just that one finds oneself feeling trapped and compulsively engaged in defensive maneuvering specifically meant at attempting to soften the impact of the abusive situation, but that it ultimately results in the same abusive predicament that the individual is trying so desperately to control; that specific quality of trauma experience led Demos to conclude that the "strategy is deeply flawed and thus they fail repeatedly, thereby experiencing painful affect" (Demos, 1998, p. 90).

In the case of Ms. G and for that matter also her mother, and perhaps less so with her sister, we see that process in operation in full gear and that explains the feeling of being stuck and finding some refuge in the protection provided by the switching of her language from primary to secondary linguistic organization of her experience. Nevertheless, she still feels the impact of her tumultuous internal world, although now formulated through a second language (Eagle, 2011; Stern, 1987). As we indicated before, this process does not appear to be within her conscious awareness because it is guided by an automatic process, the source of which is found in an evolutionary context related to a basic need to protect oneself. According to Solms and Turnbull (2002), the negative effects normally associated with an experience of trauma (i.e., fear, terror, anxiety) trigger the necessary condition for the individual to generate responses already anchored in the basic structure of the brain that get automatically mobilized to ensure the individual's basic survival. In the end, it ultimately creates organizing patterns or script structures with specific sets of associated effects that become part of response patterns and intimately ingrained in the individual's behavioral repertoire. In this context, mentation is at its minimum (if at all) (Allen & Fonagy, 2017) and the elicited emotions often become inappropriately utilized, paradoxically resulting in further threat to the individual's wellbeing.

In the case of Ms. G, her mother's presence triggers many of her old scripts that include her need to escape, run away to another country or into a new identity, acquiring and using exclusively another linguistic code. The problem is that, when affects are felt too strongly, the demands for different processing of her experience become even more important. Ms. G is adding one more component to this challenge, which is the incorporation of a different linguistic identity in which she can easily project an image of well-functioning entrepreneur whose last name will be changed through marriage; such an eventuality provides her the perfect cover, a new identity, and a new language of reference for her emotions. In the end, however, there is a danger that, in an attempt to protect herself from future traumatic conditions, she can paradoxically end up contaminating and destroying the potential for future and healthier encounters with her husband-to-be and others; this is what Thompson (1996) refers to as forging a new personal identity by opposition, or motivated by her need to distance herself from a past that it is still unprocessed.

There is another patient, Dr. E, for whom it became clear in a dream that, although highly accomplished professionally, culturally, and linguistically and seemingly well adjusted, issues of belonging still featured prominently in the recess of her mind, although not with the same intense anguish as the previous patient. Born in Venezuela, Dr. E sought treatment for a recurrent feeling of uneasiness and general feeling as *an impostor* while among her colleagues and her family. She is the younger of three children born to an immigrant family now living in the United States. In that dream,

> *Dr. E found herself looking for a previous supervisor who in the dream had his office located at the same location where she had lived in Brooklyn Heights, New York, with her ex-husband several years earlier. The office was located on the fourth floor where there were a few other therapists' offices. Although she once lived there, it took her a while to find her way around after taking different sets of stairs. As she was going through the third floor, she came across her current boss who was sitting around a small round coffee table engaged in an animated conversation with an old friend who Dr. E felt she also knew. Dr. E briefly nodded to both, with them, in turn, barely acknowledging her presence as they continued their conversation. As Dr. E was proceeding her way up to the fourth floor, she overheard her boss saying that it was a good building to live in, and that there were no minorities living there; to which the colleague who was visiting responded with a nervous smile; in Dr. E's mind, this colleague who was visiting was thinking that, perhaps, it would have been a good building for her to have considered moving in but that it was too late. That struck Dr. E as an offensive comment to make while she proceeded with her search, trying not to give much thought to it [so as not to make waves] while walking up the stairs to the fourth floor. When she was finally reaching the fourth floor, almost by happenstance, Dr. E also began to wonder how she would find her way out when finished. Eventually, she got to the last office that was located to the left at the end of the corridor where she saw a young child anxiously waiting his turn to be seen by the therapist (her friend). She was surprised and somewhat impressed that this young child of about nine years old was speaking as an adult about something that he intended to discuss with his therapist. Dr. E finally saw her friend standing by his office chair speaking with another person who was requesting (somewhat insisting) to see him; her friend looked a bit frantic trying to accommodate the request and finally offered 20 minutes gesturing "only 20 minutes" with his hands and fingers.*
>
> *The child was the son of a good colleague, well-established in her field and who was sitting next to him (her child) in the waiting room. This friend (his mother) seemed to be somewhat embarrassed but also proud of her child speaking about his therapy and divulging so openly and anxiously what he intended to speak with his therapist. Dr. E gave a brief and subtle nod of recognition and greeting to her colleague (the mother of the child) and concerned that she may resent her sudden presence, Dr. E volunteered to announce that she was just there for brief hello to Dr. Friedman (the therapist), a colleague she had not seen for quite a while. As she was waiting, Dr. E began to feel anxious about having come to the office unannounced and was then concerned that she was intruding into her colleague's busy office schedule and struggled to convince herself that it was ok to proceed, hoping that Dr. Friedman would be happy to see her come by to say hello.*

Here, we are again given a powerful opportunity to witness the internal maneuvering that even accomplished immigrant professionals find themselves struggling with, all related to feeling like the *other* and out of place and at a loss even in a building where she had lived in. The primary issue was her feeling like *an impostor* and that her colleague and her child were a lot more sophisticated and accomplished in psychological awareness than she could ever become despite her extensive training. Also prominent in the dream is her concern about making sure not to make waves about the offensive comments made by her boss to her visiting colleague that "it was a good building because there were no minorities living in the building," something she felt was a direct reference to her and as a microaggression, as a confirmation that she was indeed out of place; but also, that since it was an attractive possibility to her boss's friend, it felt to her as an affirmation that she could not trust her boss in having her best interest in mind. At the same time, there is also a sense of a lingering need for affirmation by authority figures (her supervisor) but, even that, was fraught with a great deal of anxiety. The dream was helpful in bringing to sharper focus a series of emotions that had been lingering in her for which she could not make clear sense of in her interactions with authority figures and colleagues. These were overwhelming feelings that were always present particularly when she felt that she was being directly or indirectly under scrutiny in her interactions with colleagues and supervisors, leaving her feeling physically and emotionally tired and exhausted at the end of the day. An interesting point about this case is the patient's refusal to use Spanish during her abbreviated treatment, although the issues raised in the dream pointed to core issues related to her identity as an immigrant woman with an accent who was struggling to keep her associations with individuals with a good reputation in the field, and whose friendship she felt will elevate her standing in the eyes of her colleagues.

Concluding Thoughts

It is a fascinating and intricate journey to enter the various ways language becomes so intimately involved in all aspects of the individual's cognitive and emotional life trajectory, marking, with its semantic and phonemic structures, important moments in that process. Experiences thus encoded and organized in one's language, become then permanently enshrined in memories, with language thus functioning as a container of one's lived experiences that later become the focus of the psychotherapeutic process. Enshrined in these memories are traumatic moments that are initially organized around body sensations (or in what Sullivan referred to as parataxis organizations), and later in more organized and ready-for-more conscious expressions (Sullivan, 1953); intertwined in these memories and their expressions are the specific family history that is incorporated into one's scripts that are utilized to process and deal with the challenges in one's daily life. It is that powerful link with language as an instrument for encapsulating and containing one's personal thoughts and emotions that psychoanalytic and cognitive behavioral interventions rely on in the healing process.

The importance of that connection to words as the key to getting access to the intricate content of the internal organization of lived experience was eloquently discussed in Rizzuto's (2015) erudite book on *Freud and the Spoken Word*; in this book the author provides an insightful discussion of Freud's view of speech as the key to the unconscious and, as such, anchoring the analysis of speech as an important component in psychoanalytic interventions, without neglecting other linguistic and nonlinguistic expressions that should also be attended to. It calls for attending to changes in phonemic expressions, words, and paralinguistic expressions (e.g., pressured speech, use or overuse of aahh, uhhm, amhuum; pauses, the sound emerging when clearing one's throat), the presence or absence of silence, over-verbosity or verbal paucity, etc.

Recognizing this important role of language in the cognitive process, Bucci (2021) and her team provide an empirical structure to study how personal memory is encoded in the linguistic organization and expressed through what they called "referential activity." They defined referential activity (process) as "a set of bidirectional functions that enable connection between the sub-symbolic components operating in multiple sensory channels and the discrete single channel verbal code" (p. 3). According to these authors, this process can only be understood and is based on the understanding that "human mentation involves multiple formats of thought, which are connected substantially but partially, and may operate within or outside of awareness" (pp. 3–4). It is also based on the understanding that these modes of thought include symbolic processes or "discrete representations with properties of reference and generativity." Such representations may be "images or words, and sub-symbolic components which are continuous in format and based on analogic relationships" (p. 4). Finally, it is based on the appreciation that our experiences with the world are organized "based on memory schemas, including emotion schemas organized through episodes that involve related sensory and bodily experiences with particular people in particular contexts" (p. 4).

The shifting of the language expression by Ms. G to narrating her more traumatic experience in the language and sensory structure where it was first encoded provided her with a much closer emotional connection to the original experience, as suggested by her reactions following these sessions. There were powerful opportunities, the intensity of which should be carefully monitored as it can be disorganizing to patients with poor internal resources. That should include allowing the patient to take the lead as to what language to use and, even when the therapist directly or indirectly encourages the patient to allow direct connection with these private spaces. When and how to get there should be determined by the patient's assessment of readiness.

We recognize that a more authentic and cohesive personal narrative of the past can only occur when allowing all the early emotions to be processed and integrated as a component of the self that provides meaning to one's existence in a continuous and uninterrupted sequence of all aspects of our lived experience. It allows for the progressive facing of the profound fear of being annihilated by the power of these repressed emotions in the context of a therapeutic connection with a trained professional that research findings have found to be crucial for change (Cuijpers et al., 2019; Wampold, 2015).

8

On the Neuroscientific Basis of Intersectional-Colored Trauma and Its Sequalae

Those of us working to liberate our patients from the debilitating claws of past traumatic experiences often come face-to-face with the reality that there is no easy and fast way to address this condition. Patients often come to our office holding on to the hope of receiving easy and quick pills to resolve and ease their emotional pain related to these types of experiences. We can see their agony and despair when presenting their dilemma to us as if at the mercy of something they have no power over it. Often missing from their presentation is the awareness of what the possible meaning and role of their discomforts may be and how the exploration of the nature of their different dimensions may be helpful for the ultimately healing to start. The case of Mr. T may provide us with a good illustration in this regard. He is a young light-skin man, married for several years to a darker skin woman with indigenous features whom he described as attractive and more accomplished than him. He has fathered four children, the older one with a previous relationship and still living in Nicaragua. Reportedly, he came to his first appointment complaining that he often found himself struggling with strong aggressive urges with sexual overtones, which would lead him to interact with women that he encounters in social gatherings by looking at them in ways that made them feel uncomfortable. He would go as far as seeing himself in his mind performing sexual acts with these women and being unable to stop his fantasies. For the most part, such fantasies tended to remain just that, *fantasies*, although that did not preclude his constant searching for opportunities to engage in sexual activities even outside his marriage where strong sadomasochistic quality was always in the mix.

He presented himself as having strong needs to have sex about five times a week, preferably with his wife, a situation that created great consternation for his wife who was more than satisfied with only a couple of times a week. He reported that when unable to get his sexual fix at home or through masturbation, he would visit massage parlors or would seek the services of prostitutes, particularly women of color. He described a strong preference for oral sex and a constant request to be caressed in his sexual activities by these women and prefer to seek the same prostitute for his sexual escape. Another complaint was his uncontrollable intake of alcohol and other substances, particularly during the evening hours when alone in his house before the rest of the family were to join him for dinner. This he reported as if complaining about a part of him that he has no control over and that he was so desperately trying to bring under control. He also reported to have a good job and was seemingly well-respected by his colleagues.

His wife was described as a professional woman who was juggling her multiple roles as a woman in a highly competitive white male-dominated industry and as a wife, a mother, and a daughter to her sick mother. Described as psychologically more sophisticated than him and feeling the tension growing in the family and in their relationship, she was reported to be the one who suggested that he sought professional help for himself, in addition to the work they were doing in family therapy. He reported that she was concerned with his increased use of alcohol and other substances that were affecting the family and his strong sadism that is affecting their sexual interactions.

In previous writings (Javier & Owen, 2020), we attempted to provide a scientific framework to help us recognize personal dilemmas like the one presented by Mr. T that involves a deeply ingrained position, which may be the result of a long and unexamined history of trauma. For this chapter, we hope to explore this issue further by examining the neuroscientific contexts of such development in our attempt to demonstrate the challenges in addressing these issues psychologically in our patients. Mr. T described his various obsessive maneuverings to get his hard liquor from the local store always around the same time and on the way home from work; or his being unable to stop with one drink, as he intended to, when out at a bar with coworkers or even when with those with supervisory responsibility over him. Freud (1915) referred to this position as "the stubborn adhesiveness of the libido" in the mental life that remains resistant to change and that is responsible for the patient's maintaining dysfunctional behaviors that escape psychological examinations. Since then, other explanations from evolutionary and neuroscientific investigations (Solms & Turnbull, 2002) have provided substantive support resulting in further elucidation on that very issue and that speaks to the issue of resistance to change that we find in our patients, particularly traumatized patients.

Trauma and Its Neurological and Psychic Representation

The point of departure is the recognition that patients with trauma history tend to deploy a preestablished set of rituals (personal scripts) that they have found to provide some level of relief, even if only temporary, to their internal turmoil. The other point of departure is the recognition that these rituals are automatically deployed in response to various challenges in their lives that trigger problematic feelings and that ultimately result in creating compromising situations and dysfunctional predicaments in their lives. The last point of departure is the realization that when we try to examine our patients' behavior in response to their problematic feelings, they find themselves with little or no power of control over their behavior; in the end, these individuals find themselves unwittingly recreating the same dysfunctional predicaments that they are trying to avoid, as if driven by a mysterious force, although expecting something differently (like in the case of Mr. T). This is Paul Russell's (1998a, 1998b) definition of trauma in his publications on "The Role of Paradox in Repetition Compulsion" and "Trauma and the Cognitive Function of Affects." From our perspective, we must ask the question as to what is being expressed (enacted) here; what is/are the psychic source (s) driving these reenactments, and how engrained are these in the patient's behavioral repertoire to be so automatically deployed without much mentation, if at all?

Attempts at answering these questions are found in various writings from evolutionary scholars to more psychological and psychoanalytic writings. We have addressed some of these issues in previous writings (Javier & Owen, 2020) as well, and thus we will only summarize here some of the main points made earlier. From an evolutionary perspective, several authors have advanced the view that our being in the world, our decision-making and "response style" to threatening situations, our current view of ourselves and others, and how/what we have become, are first a product of a long and transformative trajectory that is first stored and organized physiologically. These physiological organizations follow very specific parameters dictated by predetermined physiological laws whose primary function is to protect and preserve the integrity of the organism as a physical entity. We have been provided with a very sophisticated anatomical/neurological system, whose development over time has resulted in our increasingly more sophisticated capacity to respond to challenges in our environment in an automatized manner. That includes our increasingly more sophisticated capacity for abstract thinking and manipulation of our environment through more sophisticated cognitive processes related to the world of thoughts and ideas.

At the more basic level, however, even these more sophisticated structures related to cognitive processes, are guided by the same evolutionary-based system that is triggered by an experience of threat. The difference is that in the case of the latter, there is an opportunity for examination and placing automatic responses under some conscious scrutiny and control. This point was made by Warburton and Anderson (2018) who advanced a view that it is possible to alter personal scripts through systematic and sustained interventions meant to provide automatic reactions or opportunities for creating different sets of associative learning structures in the brain, something they demonstrated empirically. This is in keeping with the work of Collins and Loftus (1975) that advanced the understanding that we learn through creating a set of associations in our neural network. According to Warburton and Anderson (2018), when a new experience occurs "a node of specific neurons is set aside in the brain to recognize [this experience] . . . and to fire when it is experienced again"(p. 74). Further, when two things or events are experienced together, "the two nodes are not only activated at the same time; they start to become *neurally connected* . . . becoming strongly associated," the more often these experiences occur together (p. 74).

The fact that experiences considered similar are organized together *neurally* allows us to use them as a point of reference to understand and respond to the demands of our personal environment more efficiently. This development is made possible by the operation and is closely guided by a system that is physically centrally anchored in our nervous structure called *autonomic nervous system*, which functions as a command center, setting in motion two interrelated systems called the *sympathetic and parasympathetic nervous systems*. These two systems are automatically deployed only when situations in the external and personal environment considered threatening to our physical and psychological beings are at play. They function in concert, first to prepare the body for the required response (through the operation of the *sympathetic system*) by diverting all necessary bodily functions (e.g., blood supply, muscle tone) to address the threat at hand; this is followed by a period of normalcy (the function of the *parasympathetic system*) whenever that threat is no longer a factor; that involves the automatic shifting/returning all resources to their normal level for the benefit of the whole organism. Failure to accomplish this de-escalation of the tension normally associated with the period of threat to the organism will result in the development of various illnesses (Nevid et al., 2018/2021).

As an organism, we can only protect ourselves if we can establish and register the source and quality of these threats. The efficient operation of these systems gives us great comfort that our automatic reaction to a threat does not require a conscious decision on our part but that it is guided by a predetermined dynamism that has been effective throughout human history to ensure our safety and preservation. Part of this efficient process is the need of the organism to categorize the different qualities of the external and internal environments either as good (not threatening) or bad and likely to produce pain and discomfort (a source of threat). Warburton and Anderson (2018) indicated in this context that multiple patterns of connections are developed from our experience that is then arranged into a complex of stable links called *knowledge structure*, some of which become discrete entities known as *schemas* (p. 75). The importance of these schemas is that they contain "strongly linked thoughts, feelings, concepts, and memories related to specific aspects of experience that have in the past occurred regularly and played out similarly"; they "include knowledge about a particular facet of experience, related to attitudes, beliefs, expectations, and memories, links to typical feelings, and scripts for how to behave" (p. 75).

This mechanism is particularly active during an experience of trauma and provides us with a clear understanding of how reactions to such an experience, which are by design to be automatically deployed, can remain outside conscious awareness. It is the nature of this neurocognitive organization of traumatic experience that is at the center of what makes it so challenging, although not impossible, to eradicate the effect of traumatic memories from the individual's repertoire of responses to situations in the environment that trigger similar automatic responses.

Another component to consider in this regard relates to the fact that our personal experiences are intimately influenced by the nature and quality of our unique physical and psychological environment; that is, our socioeconomic, sociopolitical, sociocultural dynamics, or our history with intersectionality that are at play from the beginning of our involvement with the world. (For instance, someone coming from an environment of drinking, smoking, and viewing women as sexual objects of their desires may view these behaviors as a definition of a true man.) In interaction with all these components of experiences, the personal flavor of our experience is created. It is in this context that Solms and Turnbull (2002) suggested that "each of us ... has to develop his or her own individual classification of the 'good' and the 'bad' objects in the world" and "through complex interactions between our genes and the maturational environment, we develop a personal version of the world—an inner world—that is uniquely our own" (p. 278). In other words, the psychic organization described by major psychoanalytic scholars (from Freud, to Fairbairn, Winnicott, Kohut, Sullivan, Hartmann, Blanck and Blanck, and others); and the cognitive organizations described by cognitive behavioral scholars (such as Aaron Beck, Albert Ellis, David Barlow, Donald Meichenbaum, John Watson), get their specificity and personal flavors from our unique lived experience and nature and quality of our intersectionality.

On the Vicissitude of Self-Development in Traumatic Contexts

It should be of no surprise that children now exposed to war zones where their routine is frequently disturbed by bombardments and destruction of their dwellings will have their normal development characterized by these traumatic events. Such is the current situation in Ukraine and the recent earthquakes in Turkey, Syria, and Morocco that have dislodged families with their children from their home and even forced them to escape to other adjacent and friendly settings (Pistoia et al., 2018); similarly, children of immigrant families who also experience a dislodgement of their known and somewhat predictable surroundings, and are forced by circumstances beyond their control into new, unknown, and unpredictable living conditions now characterized by culturally/linguistically different environments with new rules to follow to survival in that new reality, will likely develop a psychic organization characterized by the consequences of these conditions (Zayas, 2015). If that experience also includes having to go through the ordeals of traversing dangerous territories where their physical and psychological well-being is made ever so precarious, their inner lives are likely to be characterized by these experiences. If not welcomed by the receiving country, the self-definition and the view of others emerging from these experiences will be forever anchored in their inner life, with a view of the self as located anywhere between *resilient-fragile* and *secure-overwhelmed*, and the view of the environment as located anywhere between *hostile-rejecting* and *friendly-protecting*.

On the Intimate Interplay between a Victim and a Perpetuator

Unfortunately, we have so many opportunities to examine the consequences of these types of experiences in the development of mental life with so many conditions of wars around the world. Closer to home, however, we see that same dynamic at play on various fronts: (1) In the plight of the immigrant populations that continue to challenge the border restrictions in search of better conditions for their families and now find themselves amid a political ping-pong being bused from one state to another; and (2), in the various ways our society has dealt with issues of race, gender nonconformists, linguistically and culturally diverse individuals, and the poor. It should not be much of a surprise that the self-definition of individuals characterized by intersectionality such as these and whose early (critical) experience with *the other* occurred in a society characterized by this ingrained discrimination and racism against individuals because of the color of their skin, gender, social class, religion affiliations, political persuasions, or sexual orientations, educational background (Bulhan, 1985; Gherovici & Christian, 2019; Tummala-Narra, 2021) are likely to develop a sense of self about the *others* as highly sensitive to macro- and micro-aggressive manifestations.

Similarly, it should be of no surprise that those who develop in these same societies as *doers* and *participants* in these discriminatory practices may develop a self-concept anchored in these beliefs that justify their behavior. Both trajectories in the development of self-definition in reference to the *other* are likely to be organized in the ways described by Luria (1973) and Solms and Turnbull (2002) and under the operation of an automatic system, whose organization is in the brainstem where we can find the site of our primary emotions. Because these individuals' experiences as *doers/participants* or *victims* are further cemented in each individual's psychic organization, it is likely to be then automatically triggered by perceived conditions in the environment with similar discriminatory valence. It is this automatic deployment in the absence of mentation that becomes the source of great resistance to change. It requires a constant re-examination of the appropriateness of these reactions in the context of new conditions in the interpersonal environments, which requires, in the work of Holmes (2006) and Fanon, "the dismantling of any manifestations of racism and discrimination" (Bulhan, 1985). For this to occur, it is not enough to be antiracist, it also requires a realignment of one's point of reference vis-à-vis the other, now seen as an equal partner in the journey to a different tomorrow.

Critical Moments and Trauma Development

A lot has been written about the importance of a predictable early environment during *critical moments* in the self-development and view of the world by scholars from different disciplines and theoretical and scientific persuasions (e.g., from Freud to Bowlby and colleagues, Hartmann (1939/1958), Stern (1985, 1987)). An important point in this regard is the need to examine the consequences of living in less than an expectable environment, related to the development of different attachment styles, eloquently described by Bowlby and colleagues and that is linked to the development of various psychopathologies (Bowlby, 1944; Steele & Steele, 2017). It is important to recognize that the various experiences related to different attachment styles are, by necessity, organized neurologically and ingrained in memory (within the implicit memory system) to serve as an important point of reference in our negotiation with the environment. The findings by Bowlby and colleagues (Ainsworth et al., 1978; Bowlby, 1988) and other scholars (Mikulincer & Shaver, 2017) on the development of different attachment configurations (e.g., secure, insecure, avoidant, anxious-preoccupied, resistance) within the self-organization as a function of the quality of early environments were instrumental in cementing our understanding of the way biology/physiology and psychology intersect as an organized whole.

Once established, these attachment organizations are then used as "radar" and "point of reference" to understand and guide our reactions to the environment. In a recent study, Bryant and Datta (2019) demonstrated how effective such organizations can be in dealing with distressing conditions. Those with attachment security were found to be less affected by the activation of distressing memories when compared with those with avoidant attachment tendencies. They concluded that "thinking of attachment figures during reactivation of distressing memories may decrease the distressing nature of subsequent memories" (p. 1249). They pointed to the potential application of "distressing features of memories to be modified via provision of representations of attachment figures during memory reactivation" (p. 1255) in the treatment of individuals suffering from PTSD and, in so doing, to effectively modify trauma memories in these patients. In another study by Bendezú et al. (2019), perceived attachment security was found to moderate the effects of hypothalamic-pituitary-adrenal axis (HPA) dysregulation for stress-exposed preadolescents, serving as a buffer against such dysregulation.

The debilitating effect of traumatic conditions is that they tend to derail normal development no longer characterized by "reasonably expectable environments" (Hartmann, 1939/1958). We see such possible derailments in children and families facing life and death conditions, with the continuous disruptions of their immediate environment due to wars and other political upheavals, where normalcy no longer includes a predictable outcome; or the experience facing the many immigrants' families at the mercy of unscrupulous "cayotes" where the rules of basic decency and humanity do not apply, and justifying themselves to take advantage of these individuals out of their own need for survival in their specific environment; or individuals living in countries where females are expected to be submissive and be less relevant to their male-dominated societies; or individuals growing up in a racialized society where implicit and explicit displayed of micro and blatant discriminations are present and so engrained that are often deployed with impunity and without mentation.

It should not be surprising then that people of color growing up in an environment characterized by various manifestations of different types of blatant and subtle misogynous behaviors and/or subtle and blatant racially imbued aggression and microaggression directed at them may develop highly automatized sensitivity to any manifestations where these messages may be at play (Tummala-Narra, 2021). Those delivering the "insult" may react surprised about the reactions of those receiving such an insult and are likely to respond with a dismissive statement, such as "you are too sensitive" or "I did not mean it the way you took it," or one of the many other microaggressive statements described by Sue and colleagues (2007). In keeping with our analysis, these reactions can be considered enactments of unexamined pasts that continue to create havoc in the lives of others; it creates the necessary condition for their unexamined insensitivity to be delivered without much concern of how denigrating, dismissive of one's humanity, and offensive those targeted may experience. In other words, these conditions may result in the perpetuator's insensitivity or entitlement to deliver racial insults with impunity and in hypervigilance in people of color who grow with a highly developed sixth senses to detect when such a dynamic is at play. The self-definitions emerging from these conditions are likely to impact their lives and their relationships with others differently with major consequences if left unexamined.

The Anatomy of Our Affective State

In the previous section we referred to the role of basic emotions as crucial in our understanding and responding to the world around us. In the most basic terms, we have been provided with a unique sensory structure composed of five basic senses (e.g., touch, hearing, sight, smell, and taste) originally identified by early Greek philosophers (e.g., Aristotle), each structured to provide specific information about the world around us. Recent developments are pointing to additional senses, perhaps thought to be subsumed within the previous five senses, which are operational in our body (Goldstein & Cacciamani, 2022; McClanahan & South, 2020); for instance, senses that register body temperature, direction and balance, and to regulate the carbon-dioxide content in the blood have been identified, as well as the ability to detect colors through our fingertips. Richard Youtz (a Barnard College professor) found in this regard that his blind subjects identified colors through their fingertips (Koestler, 2004).

The primary role of these senses is to bring to our awareness the changes in our physical surroundings automatically; they work in concert with our emotional systems to allow us to organize an appropriate response, depending on the nature and urgency of the perceived threat to the organism; they are responsible for (literally) pulling the alarm for action directing us to the source of the trouble. As discussed earlier, the work of Tomkins (1962, 1978) and Solms and Turnbull (2002) on the role affects and emotions provides us with an explanatory model of the unique way these emotions (particularly *fear*) function as *amplifier* to guide the nature and quality of specific responses required of us; it is a problem with emotions that propel patients to seek help and engage in all kind of defensive maneuvers to escape their effects (Solms & Turnbull, 2002; see Anna Freud [1966] and Leopold Bellak [Bellak & Goldsmith, 1984]).

According to these authors, these basic emotions that evolved throughout our evolution are now centrally anchored in our nervous systems and activate automatically to provide us with the specific information we need to respond to our environment. As explained before, encoded in these emotions are a set of recipes for actions that were effective before (although may be inappropriate for the current situation) and are anchored in memory (within the *implicit memory* structure), to be deployed in situations with similar or comparable quality. The organization of experiences with similar emotional valence as *scripts* allows us to distinguish experiences that make us feel "just good," "very good," "happy," "comfortable," "sad," "puzzled," "surprised," "afraid," or "terrorized," as well as experiences that trigger "curiosity" and "wonder." Each of us develops these scripts in unique ways as a function of our specific familial environments where we were raised, our family of origin, ecosystem, historical and political contexts, or socioeconomic and sociocultural contexts. That is, the content of these scripts will have different components of experience as a function of the extent to which the unique exposure to this multiplicity of dimensions contributed to our self-definition.

Unfortunately, to create a universal model of our mental life organization, most of the early focus of psychoanalytic thinking was primarily on the description of the development of a psychic structure assumed to have a universal appeal (Rothstein, 1985), with minimal references, if at all, to the crucial role of sociocultural contexts in this regard. We see that in Freud's (1915,1923) description of the development of the mind and its workings as driven by instinctual forces resulting in the development of personality structures around the successful/unsuccessful negotiation of Id, Ego, and Superego demands; similarly, in Sullivan's (1953) theory of personality with the tripartite personality structure of "Good Me," "Bad Me," and "Not Me"; and Fairbairn (Sutherland, 1989) and Winnicott's (1974) description of the development of the "self" as populated by "Good Object," "Bad Object," "Rejecting Object," and "Tantalizing Object" dynamic organizations emerging from the incorporation of different qualities of the early interpersonal experiences, and ultimately resulting in a psychic organization of "True" and "False self" representations in our relationship with ourselves and others (Greenberg & Mitchell, 1983).

Freud (1915, 1923) and Sullivan (1953) made clear references to the role of physiology and biological-driven forces as being the basis and foundation of all psychological development, becoming more sophisticated as our capacity to develop abstract abilities becomes possible with more sophisticated neurological structures. However, the recognition that these physiological-based forces related to our earlier development continue to exert influences on how we deal with our personal challenges, particularly when dealing with traumatic events, needs to be considered more centrally in our work with patients. It allows us to appreciate how, when we are in physical or emotional trouble, we gravitate automatically toward familiar settings and engage in familiar behavior, reaching out to family members and close friends, or any conditions that have provided us comfort earlier in our lives. It also allows us to appreciate how some patients find themselves in problematic romantic or work-related situations that have all the characteristics/qualities of situations in their earlier experiences that were painful and counterproductive (such as involvement in an abusive romantic situation after coming from a family history where alcoholism and domestic violence were present).

These are behaviors that have been explained as guided by the power of repetition compulsion, always hoping for a different outcome (Russell, 1998a, 1998b). From an evolutionary perspective, they are also the result of the operation of the deeply engrained *autonomous nervous system* described earlier. The eight basic emotions identified by Tomkins (1962, 1978) in his extensive research on the role of affects for our survival, such as "enjoyment," "interest," "distress," "anger," "fear," "startle," "disgust," and "shame"; or the four basic systems of emotions identified empirically by Solms and Turnbull (2002) (*seeking, rage, anger,* and *fear*) represent specific qualities of experience with the environment characterized by these affects. Neuroscientists have described these emotions as "organizational schemes" that provide specific information about our environment and are deployed automatically when the conditions in the external and/or internal environments call for immediate action. We are emphasizing here that we are not only referring to biologically driven conditions triggered by sensory awareness of dangerous/threatening conditions in the environment, but also reactions triggered by processes related to thoughts and memories of events that are part of our psychic organization and also associated with affects, and which may emerge in the context of our everyday experience. Again, for some, the experience of racism and discrimination may also be at play as a victim or doer. However, regardless of their sources, these reactions follow predetermined rules (to ensure quick and efficient response), with the specific mandate not only to ensure our physical safety but also our physical and psychological integrity (Luria, 1973; Nevid et al., 2018/2021; Solms & Turnbull, 2002) as determined and described by our individual experiences.

As indicated earlier, Solms and Turnbull (2002) located these reactive conditions within the control of the *limbic system* and thus considered the oldest part of the brain structure responsible for the physical survival of the living organism under the control of our *sympathetic and parasympathetic nervous systems*. However, it does not mean that the regulation of these emotions remains in this part of the brain; rather, more sophisticated parts of the brain (e.g., prefrontal and frontal sites) are also involved and are made available to us as we mature, to allow us to negotiate with the world in ways that consider external and internal considerations of appropriateness to guide our behaviors (Solms & Turnbull, 2002). These more sophisticated parts of the brain are what are not fully available to juveniles engaged in antisocial behaviors (Huss, 2014) and in adult criminals. It is as if this highly efficient circuit is compromised in those prone to impulsive behaviors (Bakhshani, 2014).

Clinical Implications

We can now return to our clinical example related to Mr. T to identify the conditions that may have contributed to his strong attraction to sadomasochistic sexuality as a vehicle for emotional survival and his general difficulty with affect regulation. An exploration of his early experience provides us with some evidence of how a series of early traumas left him quite vulnerable to feelings of abandonment and great sensitivity to feelings of rejection, but particularly a general feeling that there was something fundamentally wrong and rejecting in him. He described a mother who decided to relinquish any responsibility for him, who saw him as an imposition on her freedom and a reminder of her failed relationship with his father. He was left in the care of his extended family who treated him as a rejected and undesirable member of the family who required the pity of the whole family for his survival. He reported being under the care of an older female cousin and attaching himself to her who showed interest in him and provided him a sense of security and the feeling that he mattered. He spent a great deal of time with this cousin which included hanging around together playing and helping him with his schooling; it also included private moments when other family members were out working, or otherwise preoccupied, to allow herself to explore her sexual curiosity. Reportedly, that exploration included her teaching him how to perform oral sex on her in the secret of their home when he was very young. Although initially feeling somewhat confused that they were engaged in something that this cousin told him to keep a secret, nevertheless, he felt a special connection to this cousin and grew with a great attraction toward her who was teaching him the pleasure of the forbidden.

She was serving an important role for him at a critical moment, being that he was about five or six years old, by showing special attention in ways not exhibited by a mother who disposed of him as undesirable, a burden, and the embodiment of her intense resentment toward his father who rejected her and found her undesirable; she saw him as a reminder of her abusive, unreliable, and alcoholic husband who relinquished all responsibility as a father by abandoning the fate of the family to the care of her extended family. This cousin was then experienced as a lifesaver that gave him a recipe for survival in that family context. Thus, he learned how to keep her interested in him by becoming good at oral sex for her and eventually began to experience something pleasurable for himself as well, the source of which was not totally clear. It was a combination of feeling that he mattered and a good sensation around his mouth.

He reported feeling quite confused and puzzled when she began to show less interest in him and brought her boyfriend to the house, which in his mind became her new sex interest. He reported feeling quite despondent and angry but was also left with a recognition that there was something special about the whole experience and that there was something pleasurable for him. He was soon introduced to the feeling of euphoria when smoking cannabis with another cousin and in the context of this he experienced his fascination with how all his feelings of loneliness and despair were lifted and was left with a feeling of being at peace, soothed, and pain-free, but also at the mercy of this substance that he found irresistible.

The point that we want to emphasize at this juncture is how Mr. T's early traumas and the conditions of his early environment forced him to develop a few strategies to interact with his environment that have guided his life even into adulthood in ways predictable not only by the work of Solms and Turnbull (2002), but by most psychoanalytic and psychological theories. His current set of dilemmas finds their sources in his early trajectory of trying to survive a difficult environment whose sensorial representation became anchored in his early brain and part of his automatic nervous system, as we explained earlier. It has become intimately ingrained in his compromised psychic organization that is now guiding his relationship with himself and others, with a strong sexual and sadomasochistic overtone, with little ability to resist and apply conscious awareness. We can summarize the nature of his current dilemma as struggling with the following:

1. His tendency to sexualize his interactions with others, particularly women, and his highly sexualized dependency on them, including his wife.
2. His over-relying on orally focused dynamics (e.g., preference for leaking and sucking of the woman's breast during sex in the manner he had done with

his cousin, and the use of alcohol and cannabis, both acquiring an oral-erotic dimension).

3. His strong longing to be seen, noticed, attended to, and considered even by strangers.

4. His tendency to engage, with little ability to resist, in potentially compromising behaviors (e.g., driving under the influence; getting a sexually transmitted disease that could affect his wife) in his desperate attempt to soften the blow and find refuge, at least temporary, from the debilitated pain associated with his profound feeling of emptiness, loneliness, despair and poor/fragmented sense of self.

5. His difficulty in submitting his impulsive tendency to conscious control, guided by a progressive awareness of the core reasons for the sources of his impulsive tendencies.

Mr. T's early level of experience seems to have been developed and organized as part of what Solms and Turnbull (2002) referred to as "Primal Self," an early self-organization located in the *brainstem*, that does not have the capacity for inhibition and is guided only by basic emotions. This earliest self-organization is only concerned with the basic experience of just "being alive," considered an inherited biological given to ensure his physical survival and the inner source of awareness that is guiding his interactions with himself and others in his environment. We can see a clear parallel with Freud's (1915, 1937) view of the nature and role of instincts that he described in "Instincts and Their Vicissitudes" and "Analysis Terminable and Interminable." In this latter publication, he referred to a "constitutional strength of the instinct" as the most important "factors which are prejudicial to the effectiveness of psychoanalysis and which may make its duration interminable" (Freud, 1937, p. 221), particularly at the time of the treatment; although, he also recognized the "influence of traumas, the constitutional strengths of the instincts and the alterations of the ego" (p. 224) to be all important. It is these instinctual forces that render the individual at the mercy of the environmental demands and thus devoid of freedom, but rather dominated by the compulsion to just do and act without much examination and thus under the operation of the "repetition compulsion" mechanism (Freud, 1914/1981; Solms & Turnbull, 2002).

The fact that Mr. T finds himself unable to control his impulses suggests that the nature of his early experience with others is primarily guided by an early organization of his emotional state and under the *automatic nervous system*, the neurological representation of the mechanism of repetition compulsion; his immediate reaction to his wife's reluctance to engage in his intense sadomasochistic sexual act and that she felt uncomfortable, was that he was not doing a good job satisfying her and that he should try harder (a reenactment of the early scenario with his cousin who lured him into performing oral sex on her and then, inexplicably, pushing him aside, leaving him confused).

There was the beginning of some awareness on his part regarding possible reasons why his behavior was creating problems for him with his wife. That came about in response to an interpretation of the various ways he was obsessed with deriving sexual satisfaction even from prostitutes. Such behavior was framed as his tendency to view women primarily as a sexual objects of his intense urge for sex that ultimately resulted in stripping them of their own humanity and any expression of their personal journey. He made a connection in that the possible reason his wife was avoiding him and did not share the same desire for the frequency of sex was that she may be feeling that he was just viewing her also primarily as an "object of his sexual desire," depriving her of her own humanity, and imbuing in her sexual desires that were not in her but likely belonging to someone else (his cousin).

Another component that emerged as a possible source of the intensity may have to do with his view of her with darker skin and viewed in his culture as having extraordinary sexual desire. In the end, he ended up using the preconceived notion of Black women in his cultural context to justify the appropriateness of how to satisfy his own sexual desire. In recent sessions, we have some evidence that he is becoming aware that there is something else driving his condition when he recently communicated that "I am aware that it has to do with something else" and "just need to find out without going along with it." He also is beginning to recognize and is requesting the active "help" of his wife (a search for a more actively-involved mothering figure) to curtail his need for alcohol by putting limits to his intake.

The great challenge in working with this patient has to do with the nature of the work that is necessary and that must focus on several fronts; it should include the following to provide a counter to his strong compulsive tendency:

1. The first front is helping the patient recognize that his previous attempts to soften the blow of his psychic pain are not working and have become counter-productive. In this context, help him identify some of the reasons.
2. It should include a detailed exploration of the range of feelings, the specific triggers for his reactions, and help identify some of the possible explanations of the reasons for their intensity.
3. Concerning his interaction with his wife, we should explore his complicated view of her as darker-skinned woman assumed to have insatiable sexual desire and a tremendous capacity to provide care and emotional support for him. Here, his need to objectify her as a sexual object who is imbued with the capacity for nurturance suggests both admiration and envy at play, as well as fear of disappointing her and the lingering possibility that she will end up rejecting him. These are all dynamics related to his first sexual encounter with his cousin who ended up rejecting him.
4. It should include helping him make a detailed inventory during the sessions of his attempts to curtail his expressions of these feelings; it may also involve giving him specific assignments to use journaling to force more awareness of his activities closer to the time when they are happening, with the task of focusing on what was happening with him in terms of feelings and thoughts (or triggers) that were involved. This focus is meant to help his previous impulsive activities to become more under the control of conscious awareness both in terms of possible sources and the nature of the intensity. It should also include helping him identify areas that have worked or are working well for him.

5. Finally, helping him develop specific strategies that may encourage the progressive transformation of his responses to his old impulsive tendencies with new and specific strategies that allow a recognition of the psychic sources being expressed. This is what Freud (1905) refers to as the process of sublimation or the process of transforming an old destructive way into a more personally helpful and less compromising manner.

It is important to keep in mind, however, that being aware does not translate necessarily into true insight as for true insight to occur it also requires actively working toward changing the behavior. As Sedler (1983) indicated summarizing the view of working through by Freud, it involves "recognizing resistances (insight) and overcoming resistances (change)" (p. 73). For Gil (1988), the task of psychoanalytic work is ultimately to help patients to reengage with their personal environment "by focusing the interpretations not only on transference and reconstruction, but also on the determinants currently affecting the patient's relationships beyond transference" (p. 535).

Where Can We Go from Here?

Our decision to delve into this discussion about the clinical material described earlier is meant to highlight that these automatic reactions may be linked to early interactions with people in our external environment where a relationship or "momentary state of the core self in relation to its concurrent surround of objects" was established, resulting in the development of a "unit of consciousness" (Solms & Turnbull, 2022, p. 276). These authors referred to this unit of consciousness as a "self-state," or "a moment of awareness" (p. 276), where the individual comes to an important realization that he/she needs to interact with things/people in their immediate surroundings in ways to secure their survival (e.g., need for food when hungry, shelter when cold, and care in general). According to these authors, the earliest the experience that sets in motion one's development, the more likely it is organized at the visceral level and established in a sensory mode (within the *procedural memory structure*); such an organization allows for quick deployment when called for and gives rise to a "self-state" characterized by these dynamics. Solms and Turnbull (2002) locate these types of representational contents in the brain structures that are "dedicated to the reception, analysis, and storage of information about the world" and include a coupling of "a momentary state of the core self in relation to its concurrent surround of objects" (p. 279); such a coupling makes the relationship with the world as "the essence of consciousness" and affirms the fact that our "inner needs can only be satisfied by things that exist beyond ourselves" (p. 279). Freud (1905) describes this process at the most fundamental level when recognizing in his description of psychosexual development that it is important to include a relationship with others outside oneself for the full fulfillment of the sexual drive to be possible. It is in this context that he speaks about the concept of "perversion" as a detour regarding the best conditions to satisfy the ultimate "aim" of those instinctual drives, which should be the preservation of the species.

Putting aside the controversy of that being a requirement, perversion in this context refers to the moving away from the need to include others in mutual exchange in pursuing one's sexual satisfaction. The case of fetishism, frotteurism, voyeurism, exhibitionism, and other paraphilias are examples of the consequences of a fundamental detour regarding the ultimate aim. In a more general way, it is possible to refer to perversion as any detour from our primary realization that we need the other to survive. This issue was amply illustrated in the influential work of Sullivan (1953), Fairbairn (Greenberg & Mitchell, 1983), Winnicott (1974, 1986a, 1986b, 1988), and Aron (1996) where disorders were described as an inability to develop meaningful interactions/relationships with others resulting in conditions ranging from neurotic to borderline, to psychotic-like conditions.

There are several components of an ideal treatment for individuals with a history of trauma and whose interactions with themselves and others are greatly compromised by the automatic deployment of crippling reactions. There are various approaches to treatment interventions that have primarily focused on specific changes in behaviors and cognitions related to traumatic events. For instance, eye movement desensitization and reprocessing (EMDR), which involves eye tracking of visual target while holding images of the traumatic experience in mind (Nevid et al., 2018/2021), has been found to produce relief but we still have limited knowledge of its underlying mechanism of action (Landin-Romero et al., 2018). Other treatments focus exclusively on working with cognitive distortions and behavioral changes (Foa, 1997). It is clear, however, that because of the multiple issues that are frequently at play with a trauma profile individual, the ideal treatment should include multiple prongs and consider conditions that may have made this individual vulnerable to future traumatic events. From that perspective the ideal treatment should include direct and specific interventions to alleviate the immediate debilitating effect of trauma conditions, but also to make sure to scaffold such interventions in a systematic and careful exploration of factors that create and fuel its current presentation.

Psychoanalytic conceptualization provides us with the best model to accomplish such an important scaffolding as it focuses primarily on the following: (a) on the examination of conditions, unconscious/out of awareness motivations; (b) factors that are likely to be directly/indirectly relevant to understanding the patient's traumatic reaction; (c) emotional and cognitive factors and unconscious/unformulated ways that trauma patients respond to triggers in their external and internal environments and likely to be influencing their maintenance of the trauma manifestation (Allen & Fonagy, 2017); and (d) it provides the most insightful opportunities for patients to change/curtail the effect of their *knowledge structures* through the evaluation of their perceptions in the context of transference and countertransference manifestations, considered as powerful and vivid displays of how one's internal organization gets acted out/enacted in the here and now during the therapy session in real time. The emphasis that only with the emergence of conscious awareness and control of our unconscious emotions is cure possible, is one of the primary tenets of psychoanalytic conceptualization. Support of this view can be found in the work of Koch and associates who concluded that it is not the event itself "the most important predictor of PTSD but that individual characteristics and perception of the event are the most relevant factors" (cited by Javier & Owen, 2020, p. 21), in addition to the nature, quality, and intensity of the trauma event. With that as a framework, we are suggesting that the ideal and best intervention for trauma experience should consider the following, some of which were listed in reference to the treatment of Mr. T:

(1) Recognize that reactions that are triggered automatically by various conditions in the external and internal conditions can only be explained by examining more carefully the nature of the feelings triggered by these interactions. Since it is likely that these patients will react equally strongly to a therapist's intervention manifested as transference reactions, we should make use of such an opportunity to demonstrate the distortion in perception that may have triggered the reaction. I am reminded of a patient who responded with a violent verbal outburst to a question asking him if he had any sense as to what his supervisor was asking of him? In his outburst he screamed "Why are you asking me that question?" "Why are you taking their side?" "They are just a bunch of incompetent morons, without college education." I may have tapped inadvertently into old emotional wounds of traumatic nature.

(2) Recognize that such reactions in patients suggest *"the presence of tremendous fear,"* for which they felt compelled to respond defensively with violent outbursts in their attempt to repel the threat. Exploring the nature of the fears and other emotions in this context may be instructive and helpful to reach a more compressive understanding of the multiple emotional dilemmas at play and contextualize/anchor these emotions within their lived experiences.

(3) Engage in mapping as many situations as possible along this quality of relating and responding to difficult emotions. Also, identify specific situations when the patient responded differently and more appropriate, and examine the specific components of these interactions as well, as they may help explain the differences in their reactions in terms of the sources of the feelings generated.

(4) Be cognizant and careful about not being judgmental in our inquiry but rather anchor it in the recognition of the patient's lived experience. This is particularly important when a patient's experiences differ from our own regarding being victims of discrimination related to race, gender, age, sexual orientation, socioeconomic situation, educational levels, or cultural and linguistic backgrounds. For instance, the patient referred to in number 1, also included as part of his outburst phrases such as "fat, black, incompetent moron, who got the supervisory position because of personal connection," when he felt criticized and brought to tasks by the supervisor. On another occasion, when he felt attended to and stroked by the supervisor, he would report praising this same supervisor with such comments as "she truly knows what she is doing," "I needed to get her opinion and she was helpful," something that he would report with a sense of having been attended to. In his case, we have uncovered a few experiences of being rejected by his own ethnic group, feeling like

the black sheep of his family, and constantly being attracted to women of color as emotional partners.

(5) Once we have been successful in anchoring their reactions as emerging from pre-established scripts that were appropriate and/or inappropriately deployed, we can then assess the specific consequences in the various situations and various people in their lives.

(6) Provide a detailed explanation of what it will take to minimize the presence of their dysfunctional reactions by anchoring their experience as having been shaped by unexamined feelings which may have served a very appropriate function before, but which are now creating more problems for them in being able to attain their ultimate goal.

(7) Design specific strategies to help these patients monitor their reactions using journaling and giving them specific tasks to help them advance in their ability to manage their emotions while outside of treatment setting.

(8) Utilize group-based intervention to provide these patients with an opportunity for external feedback loop of how they are coming across to others, while also working individually on identifying the sources of their reactions in the context of their lived experience; it should also include an opportunity for assessing the accuracy/appropriateness of their responses to others in terms of their assessment of the possible distortions of perceptions regarding others' motivations for what they do or say. According to Warburton and Anderson (2018), people prone to respond aggressively tend to have poor reappraisal skills of their own contributions to a situation.

These types of interventions are meant to provide an opportunity to address inaccurate and inappropriate *knowledge structures* and work on and strengthen the patients' cognitive/affective abilities. It also emphasizes the findings that brain plasticity and the ability to acquire new ways of dealing with one's surroundings remains viable even in an aged brain that has been found to retain a high level of plasticity (Jessberger & Gage, 2008).

Conclusion

It was our intention in this chapter to provide a general overview of the neural basis of our emotions and the various ways they are intimately involved in who we are and what defines us physically and psychologically. In this context, we discussed findings from evolutionary and neuroscientific scholars which have provided a clear description of this process and that has resulted in "who" and "what" we become to ourselves and others. All our emotional repertoire (or basic emotions) has been specifically developed in response to the demands of our internal and external environments, serving as an important organizing structure. This process was eloquently elucidated, described, and explained by Tomkins (1962, 1978), Solms, and Turnbull

(2002) in their various publications which have provided us with the language to describe such a process; particularly important is the fact that these emotions are anchored in an automatic reaction loop that does not require mentation and is likely to be activated in individuals with a history of trauma. It is this unique quality of emotions associated with traumatic experiences that makes treatment of trauma so challenging. Nevertheless, recognizing that neuroplasticity is still present in older adults, and guided by findings that it is possible to improve the capacity to place one's behavior under conscious control, we made specific treatment recommendations meant to establish new associative links that foster the deployment of one's behavior based on personal awareness of their appropriateness and less under the automatic nervous system control. This is accomplished through a detailed assessment/exploration of the individual actions in terms of motivation and emotions associated with these actions. In this context, some specific tasks were recommended meant to create the condition that will make it more likely for someone to do well in an environment different that his/her previous background.

On Inherent Psychological Factors in Some Criminal Behaviors

From the very beginning of civilization, a fascination with the dark side of human experience has captured the attention of philosophers, social and political scientists, and behavioral scientists. The difficulty in finding a reasonable explanation of someone's behavior that falls outside the parameters of what we consider normal has contributed to delegating such behaviors to a manifestation of pure evil. In psychology, the word *psychopathy* has been used to categorize such behaviors (Cleckley, 1941; Hare, 1996), with the additional question as to whether there is any hope for rehabilitation and change in the motivational path normally ascribed to these individuals. Although treatment methods are still in need of further refinement for this population, we remain fascinated as a society in trying to understand "the criminal mind". This is demonstrated by the ever-growing media-produced programs such as television shows like *The Criminal Mind* and *Dateline*, podcasts like "My Favorite Murder," and movies such as *The Silence of the Lambs* that focus on sexual predators, criminals with sadistic and cannibalistic preferences, and serial killers.

The lingering question of the extent to which depravity and the notion of pure evil and sadism can dwell in the mind and souls of our fellow human continues to be triggered by seemingly never-ending broadcasts of yet another assault and killing of a store owner/clerk for a few dollars; or the news of an elderly Asian woman or man being punched just because they belong to different ethnic groups, as occurred during the height of the COVID-19 epidemic. We suspect that it is this lingering question, the curiosity, and desire to understand these types of behaviors that attract many of us to true crime stories. Televised courtroom proceedings, such as Court TV, bring viewers into the real-life courtrooms and provides the opportunity to see the ins and outs of crimes committed firsthand, including the process of witnesses being deposed and defendants testifying on their behalf. We no longer have to imagine the crime as depicted in movies because detailed visual information is frequently depicted in these televised proceedings. For instance, a recent blow-by-blow trial proceeding was shown on Court TV with defendant Alex Murdaugh. His trial captured the attention of the media and nation alike, as he is someone who had a seemingly successful practice as a lawyer and who comes from a prominent legal family in South Carolina that has had tremendous influence in that legal community for years. He was described as having a long history of engaging in legally questionable behaviors and manipulating the legal system to his advantage. His long-standing criminal activities finally caught up with him and he was found guilty of killing his wife and one of his sons on June 7, 2021, with the supposed motives of attempting to cover other misdeeds. Other possible crimes ascribed to him included embezzling funds from his legal firm, further portraying him as a man who did not feel the law applied to him and his family. He was described, and he described himself, as a chronic liar who lied his way through many situations assisted by a legal system that gave him cover and the benefit of the doubt. This may have been out of deference to the prestige and power the family had exercised in that legal community for years, or for fear of what further harm he could do under the cover of the law. His depravity went as far as maneuvering to represent his housekeeper's family in an accident that occurred at his own residence which resulted in her death. Murdaugh then kept most of the insurance money to himself, only giving a very small portion to the woman's family. The most recent legal proceeding involving the death of his wife and son was a lengthy and sensationalized trial that attracted media outlets from all over the world to witness aspects of the trial, such as his only remaining son testifying on behalf of his father. Hundreds of onlookers camped outside the court daily to secure one of the few seats available inside. The fascination even extended to several people interested in getting a piece of "murderabilia" of items from the Murdaugh's home sold recently at an auction to compensate his victims.

We were equally fascinated by several other cases that provided us with a peek at possible motivating factors behind their crimes. One such case recently adjudicated was that of a young man, Nicholas Cruz, who pleaded guilty to killing 14 students and three staff members, and injuring 17 others at Parkland School in Florida, a school that he had attended but from which he had been suspended; he was described as someone with untreated serious mental condition (Washington Post Staff, 2018), including previous cruelty to animals, serious school problems, a pervasive fascination with guns, and abusive relationship toward his adopted mother.

Finding motivational factors to explain the reasons for the next two crimes is more challenging. The first one is that of "Doomsday Mother" Lori Vallow a woman convicted of having her two children from her previous marriages killed by her brother under the belief that they were "zombies." Her current husband Chad Daybell, described as a Doomsday Prophet, is also accused (and now waiting for trial) of being involved in the killing and disposing of their bodies, as well as the killing of his previous wife, for seemingly the same belief of her becoming a zombie.

Finally, the case of 16-year-old Aiden Fucci belongs to a different category of crime. Recently convicted of killing 13-year-old Tristyn Bailey with 114 stab wounds, Fucci was given a life sentence with a possibility of parole after 25 years because of his age at the time of the crime. Had he been older, he would have been eligible for the death penalty sentence because of the cruelty, coldness, and premeditation of the crime. There was nothing the court could find that could explain or mitigating factors involved in his killing, only that he wanted "to feel what was like to kill someone" and carefully lured this young girl into her death to achieve this. His demeanor during the court proceeding, including during sentencing while the judge was laying out the rationale for the sentence about to be imposed, was of someone deprived of emotions as if in an altered state of mind (Court TV, 2023).

Is There a Reasonable Explanation for Criminal Behaviors?

Many attempts have been made to provide an explanation for engaging in such behaviors, seen as aberrant and representing the dismantling of all the parameters or laws created over centuries to curtail behaviors considered destructive and counter-productive to the benefit of our society. This view of criminality has been influenced by the experience of fear and terror generated by these acts, which has subsequently resulted in creating prisons to give us the illusion of being protected from becoming victims of these criminal acts (McCormick, 1950). An often-referred-to quote in this regard, whose actual origin dates back to earlier thinkers, is the proposition espoused by Machiavelli in his 1513 treaty "The Prince" where he concluded that, in the end "*Homo homini Lupus est*" (a man is a wolf to another man) in our relationship to others and thus guided by the principle that "the end justifies the means," and that "no man can ultimately be trusted" (Gardner, 2010, p. 2); although not intended to explain criminality, such a view may nevertheless provide an important perspective of what may be operating particularly in criminal minds. In this same vein, the philosopher Hobbes viewed men (humanity) as "predisposed to violent action" and hence the need to create/impose conditions through laws in the society "in order to prevent the destruction of man in an anarchic society" (Gardner, 2010, p. 2).

From a psychological perspective we are left with the question of how we are to make sense of the crimes committed by Alex Murdaugh, Nicholas Cruz, Lori Vallow, and Aiden Fucci? They can be considered an aberration of a normal process in our development as humans, one that is not supposed to happen and, if it happens, it must be the result of an abnormal development that can only be construed as rooted in a disease of the brain. That was the view of Wilhelm Griesinger, a German physician who argued that abnormal behaviors must be seen in that light (Nevid et al., 2018/2021). Such a view was seen as an important departure from earlier perspectives that construed these types of behaviors as a result of demonic possession and witchcraft. This biological view was supported by the experience of many in the medical profession of witnessing bizarre behavioral manifestations in individuals who were found to suffer from syphilis (a bacterium that invades the brain). Such a disease causes primarily personality and mood changes in their patients, as well as affecting memory functioning and judgment. Considering that all symptoms disappeared when given penicillium (Nevid et al., 2018/2021) provided an important insight as to the true causal link for these disorders. It was not until the work of Ribot (1891) that we began to witness a solid movement toward a more systematic study of behaviors that were considered abnormal. He saw the study of mental illnesses or diseases, as "the morbid derangement of the organism," and further elaborated on this concept in his books on *The Diseases of Personality* (1891), *Diseases of the Will* (1895), and *Diseases of Memory: An Essay in the Positive Psychology* (1896) (cited by Makari, 2008). In these writings, Ribot provided the necessary scientific foundation for studying these phenomena in terms of their biological and neurological sources. However, the work of Charcot (Strachey, 1893) was the first to provide the necessary ingredients for a true paradigm shift in that he demonstrated that a seemingly medical condition could be created by psychological processes. He created or removed paralyzes that were physically crippling the person's functions (such as hysterical blindness and paralysis of the limbs) through hypnotic suggestions demonstrating that other processes were at play in creating debilitating conditions; in essence, the disease of the mind can also affect the person's overall physical condition. It is this history where we see the seminal work of Freud (1894/1896, 1915, 1923, 1926) in providing us with the first psychological model of the mind and a sophisticated view of the different psychological forces at play in the development of these types of behaviors. We will return to Freud's contributions in explaining the dark side of human behaviors later in this chapter.

A Psychological Explanatory Model of Criminal Behavior

More specifically related to criminal behaviors, we can see early attempts at encouraging the application of psychological principles to explain criminal behaviors. With his seminal book *On the Witness Stand*, Hugo Munsterberg (1908) introduced the first psychological treatment on the subject, further refined by Hervey Cleckley (1941) in his book on *Mask of Sanity* and by the work of Robert Hare (2001). Sixteen specific categories of behavior were identified by Cleckley (1941) as descriptive of criminal behaviors, particularly behaviors with a psychopathic overtone (see Textbox 9.1), which then provided the necessary framework for the development of the first and most durable system to categorize criminal behaviors (the Hare's Psychopathy Checklist or PCL and the further revised version PCL-R) as resulting from very specific conditions.

The PCL and PCL-R allow us to group criminal behaviors into two distinct categories or factors based on their presentations: For Factor 1, characteristics related to interpersonal and affective qualities involved in criminal behavior are included, while for Factor 2 he included characteristics related to a socially deviant/antisocial lifestyle (e.g., early behavioral problems and parasitic, impulsive/poor behavioral controls) that are found to have early manifestations during adolescence (see Table 9.1) (Huss, 2014).

But it is the categorization of primary versus secondary psychopathic traits that provides us with the best description to identify psychopathic behaviors as coming from two different sources: *Primary psychopathy* is usually found to result from some inherent deficits and is characteristic of prototypical psychopathy, antisocial acts, irresponsibility, lack of empathy, superficial charm, and absence of any anxiety. By contrast, *secondary psychopathy* is usually found in a relationship with factors such as low intelligence, some sort of social disadvantage, and the presence of impulsivity that is normally driven by anxiety (Huss, 2014). The issue with the

Textbox 9.1.
Unique Characteristics Describing Psychopathy

Sixteen characteristics in the clinical profile of psychopathy:

1. Superficial charm and good intelligence
2. Absence of delusions and other signs of irrational thinking
3. Absence of nervousness
4. Unreliability
5. Untruthfulness and insincerity
6. Lack of remorse or shame
7. Inadequately motivated antisocial behavior
8. Poor judgment and failure to learn from experiences
9. Pathological egocentricity and incapacity for love
10. General poverty in major affective reactions
11. Specific loss of insight
12. Unresponsiveness in interpersonal relations
13. Fantastic and uninviting behavior with drink (sometimes without)
14. Suicide is rarely carried out
15. Sex life is interpersonal, trivial, and poorly integrated
16. Failure to follow any life plan

Table 9.1. **Factors Found in Two Different Types of Psychopathy**

Factor 1	Factor 2: Socially Deviant/ Antisocial Lifestyle	Additional Factors
• Glibness/superficial charm • Grandiose sense of self-worth • Pathological lying • Conning/manipulative • Lack of remorse or guilt • Shallow affect • Callous/lack of empathy • Failure to accept responsibility for own actions.	• Need for stimulation/ proneness to boredom • Parasitic lifestyle • Poor behavioral controls • Early behavioral problems • Lack of realistic, long-term goals • Impulsivity • Irresponsible • Juvenile delinquency • Revocation of conditional release	• Promiscuous sexual behavior • Many short-term marital relationships • Criminal versatility

DSM-5 diagnostic categories is that it does not recognize psychopathy, and it diffuses the seriousness of psychopathy as a condition motivated by different sources. We recognize that it does include psychopathic items such as lying, cheating, and stealing as part of antisocial personality disorder (ASPD), with the psychopathy criteria included in that context described in terms of behavioral and interpersonal/affective characteristics. We find, however, that antisocial personality disorder diagnosis does not provide sufficient clarity of the dangerousness that is often found under psychopathy when characteristics listed under Factor 1 are prevalent. Psychopathy as a category is found to be narrower and much more specific than ASPD, with only 15–30% of individuals categorized as ASPD that are also found to suffer from true psychopathy (Huss, 2014).

Additionally, there have been some concerns as to the best way to determine the presence of antisocial behaviors and psychopathy among diverse ethnic, racial, and cultural populations, considering the overrepresentation of this population in the legal system, particularly among incarcerated individuals (Leidenfrost & Antonius, 2020; Stevens & Morash, 2014; Western et al., 2021). According to Leidenfrost and Antonius (2020), "African Americans and Hispanics were incarcerated at six to seven times the rates of White offenders . . . with African Americans making up approximately 40% of the total incarcerated population" (p. 85). These authors also noted widespread trauma histories among that population, with trauma events occurring before incarceration, a point also highlighted by Garbarino (2015) and by Nesi et al. (2020). While we recognize that not all incarcerated individuals suffer from psychopathy, we do make the assumption that most of these individuals have or are assumed to have been engaged in antisocial behaviors. The Hare's Psychopathy Checklist referred to earlier has functioned as the standard measure in this regard and is widely accepted by the scientific community; nevertheless, we are still in need of further refinements in these assessment tools to make them more sensitive to assess the diverse populations, particularly regarding cultural and socioeconomic contexts.

In his 2014 book, Huss noted a series of attempts at determining rate of psychopathy among different gender, ethnic, and cross-cultural samples and highlighted the tremendous challenges normally associated with such an effort. He noted the inconsistency of findings depending on the instruments and the nature of samples (e.g., community versus adjudicated samples), leading him to conclude that we can only make tentative pronouncements in this regard. A similar conclusion was also made by Verona et al. (2010) earlier when summarizing the status of empirical findings in that regard. With this caveat in mind, we will now highlight some of these findings reported by Verona et al. (2010). They reported that there is a higher prevalence and mean scores of psychopathy among the North American sample as compared to the European sample suggesting that the rate of individuals likely to be engaging in behaviors with psychopathic overtone is found to be higher in the United States, as measured by PCL-R checklist, when compared with samples from other countries. The only reasonable conclusion that we can derive from these findings is not that there is a higher percentage in the United States in comparison to other countries, but that the measures utilized and originally developed for the United States may not be reliable and accurate for use in other countries without some modifications. Because psychopathy, when present, is found to be a strong predictor of violence and recidivism across-culturally, with the cognitive and emotional deficits found in this population to be present across different countries (Huss, 2014; Verona et al., 2010), it is crucial that we get a better sense of the accurate rate of psychopathy in our midst.

Additionally, no sufficient evidence has been found that African Americans have higher scores of psychopathy traits than Caucasians. What has emerged, particularly when comparing the rate of psychopathy among the young population, is that "the symptoms of the disorders may be expressed differently, more difficult to assess, and less stable in childhood and adolescence than in adulthood" (Verona et al., 2010, p. 320). Ethnic differences have been found in that ethnic/minority youth are more likely to score as slightly elevated on measures of psychopathic tendencies, such as callous-unemotional, narcissism, impulsivity, and conduct problems, as compared with nonminority youths in the community and clinic-referred samples. This finding is in keeping with the assumption of criminality reported and feared by many Black youths when in interactions with law enforcement personnel; it may also be driving the likelihood of minority youths ending up incarcerated (Leidenfrost & Antonious, 2020).

Finally, research findings regarding gender differences among the youth population in community samples that reported boys score higher in impulsivity and conduct problems, and are likely to show a more callous-unemotional picture than girls, is also in need of further exploration. For instance, when looking at incarcerated youth, higher scores in impulsivity and conduct problems were found among the girls, but not callous-unemotional qualities. Instead, in one study reported by Verona and associates (2020), girls were found to be less likely to show problems with interpersonal and emotional traits. This means that they were less likely to come across as arrogant and deceitful; even so, no differences between males and females were found along these dimensions in another study (Verona et al., 2010), which suggested instead that these two groups tended to be similar in impulsiveness, arrogance, and deceitfulness in some contexts.

These inconsistencies in research findings led Zuckerman (2003) to conclude that any differences between African-American, Native-American, Hispanic, and European-American groups in antisocial behavior "seems to be more a function of social class, historical circumstance, and their position in Western society rather than racial genetics" (p. 1463). From our perspective, although we have highlighted the serious problems with determining the extent to which level of psychopathy may be present among diverse populations, it does not minimize the recognition that psychopathic behaviors, when present, can be organized along primary versus secondary psychopathy dimensions, as discussed earlier in this chapter. This is important because the presence of traumatic histories has been found to characterize the criminal histories of incarcerated individuals (Leidenfrost & Antonious, 2020), the recognition of which may help contextualize these behaviors.

A View of Criminality in Psychoanalytic Contexts

When we try to classify the cases listed earlier in this chapter along the categories suggested by Hare and others, we encounter a bit of challenge with Alex Murdaugh.

His overall profile is that of a psychopath primarily characterized with Factor 1 qualities; he matched this profile until he was convicted of killing his wife and one of his children. This is a very unlikely act in someone with a psychopathic profile, as primary psychopaths are more likely to victimize strangers (Huss, 2014). They are also more prone to commit more crimes than those suffering from ASPD, with those crimes being more instrumental or planned (referred to as *impulsively instrumental* by Hart & Dempster, 1997), as compared to reactive (Huss, 2014). From the perspective of whether there are mitigating circumstances that may be contributing to the antisocial behavioral maneuvering that characterized his overall behavior with others, we have not found any. What emerges is a sense of entitlement in his overall behavior, of engaging in these deviant acts just because he could, to satisfy a narcissistic need. Similar comments regarding the presence of narcissism but also of sadism can be made in the case of Aiden Fucci, where the only reason found for his murdering the young woman was just for the thrill of it, "to know how it feels to see someone die." This blind homicidal discharge was described by Freud (1928) as boundless egoism and the presence of a strong destructive urge. Subsequent explanatory models by several scholars (Kernberg, 1984; Meloy & Shiva, 2007) also viewed the role of narcissism as an important focus of analysis in explaining criminal behaviors. For Meloy and Shiva (2007), for instance, such behavior can only be explained by recognizing that these criminal acts are characteristics "fueled by an absence of emotional attachment to others: the bond that keeps most people from destroying those whom they love" (p. 335), or feel they cannot obtain. In the case of Nicholas Cruz, although we find more mitigating circumstances at play (as seen in secondary psychopaths), his act was premeditated, calculated, and planned, all characteristics normally found more prominently in primary psychopaths; again, suggesting the presence of some pathological narcissism and sadism at play. The case of Lori Vallow and Chad Daybell is a bit more complicated. Lori's destruction of her children requires rejection or expulsion and disavowal of something very personal and whose continuous presence creates a constant reminder that becomes too painful to bear, with the ultimate fear of the annihilation of the self. Thus, by projecting and expelling these disavowed aspects of herself onto her children and then depriving them of their humanity by calling them zombies, Lori created the necessary justification for their destruction and the assumed attainment of her sought-after purification from all murderous/destructive feelings, toxicity, and evilness residing in her. Again, suggesting the presence of psychopathy with a strong pathological narcissism overtone characterized by murderous and destructive impulses that were unleashed against those she considered obstacles to her ultimate personal gratification. That is because by destroying those she considered unworthy she would be opening the way to being considered one of the selected 144,000 to be saved for a blissful afterlife mentioned in the Biblical scripture and literally endorsed by her cult. What has most recently emerged is that the motivation for all these crimes may have been guided ultimately by the oldest destructive forces known to humans: greed, power, and lust. Her crime may be considered as ultimately due to the presence of a psychotic process, but was clearly fueled by a pathological narcissistic condition characterized by megalomania and strong delusion of grandeur. We saw that in full display at the sentencing phase when given an opportunity to speak; she spoke about her special gift of being able to witness and experience how much at peace in the afterlife were the people that she was found guilty in orchestrating their deaths.

The Role of Trauma in Criminal Behaviors

Freud's (1915) view on the role of instincts in the human condition could be construed as one of the first attempts to provide a possibly explanatory model for understanding criminal behaviors when he wrote about the inherently destructive nature related to instinctual forces in all of us and that requires the taming of these forces to ensure our preservation as a society. In this context he makes references to the process by which sublimation of these forces becomes an essential accomplishment in humanity to insure our productive engagement with the external worlds and one another. The role of trauma is front and center in his conceptualization when explaining the process of symptom formation as a derailment of the normal process caused by traumatic events (1894/1896). He viewed it as a crucial ingredient in the development of psychopathology and later chronicled by Bowlby (1944, 1969) in his work on the different development of attachment disorders possible, resulting from a direct consequence of the quality and nature of trauma experienced during the critical developmental years. As described in other chapters in this book, this perspective is based on the recognition that under the best of circumstances, we come into this world provided with the necessary biological and physiological equipment to negotiate our interactions with ourselves and the world around us to ensure our physical and psychological survival. The work of Margaret Mahler and her colleagues (1975, 1979a, 1979b) provides us with detailed descriptions of the process through which we progress physiologically and psychologically as we mature and develop the capacity to organize, categorize, and remember our experiences with our environment in ways that will ensure our survival. Their research chronicled the ultimate result of that process with our development as psychological beings who are secure, integrated, independent, empathic, relatable, and able to remember how best to interact with our world with mutuality of purpose.

More specifically related to the development of criminality and to the role of trauma in some criminal behaviors, Garbarino (2015) provides us with ample examples of criminals he assessed in his book *Listening to Killers*, some of whom were found guilty of capital crimes, and for whom severe trauma during critical developmental years was front and center in their lives. He highlighted the level of serious vulnerability and fear that still resided in the psyche of these individuals. In this context, he described his work with a 30-year-old inmate by the name of Danny Samson, who was already condemned to two death sentences; Samson was described as a very dangerous and menacing man with bulging muscles and tattoos, and whose hands and feet have to be shackled and a chain anchoring his belt to a bolt on the floor, and that he required the presence of six correction officers surrounding him when in court (Garbarino, 2015). He had an extensive record of involvement with the criminal system since the age of 15, including a history of repeated violent assaults on other inmates and the murder of another. After reviewing his life history,

Garbarino (2015) described him as "a very damaged person, emotionally, morally, and spiritually" (p. 1), but also someone who had trouble being alone in the dark. In response to a question, he indicated that he often finds himself crying "himself to sleep at night," a revelation that led Garbarino to conclude that "inside this big, scary, dangerous man is a frightened and hurt little child" (p. 1).

Garbarino (2015) was not referring to a single trauma found in many of the criminals he assessed but the persistent presence of traumatic conditions in their lives. He found that it is "an accumulation of traumas and other risks factors . . . with little in the way of positive developmental assets to help compensate for the assaults on their psyches" (p. 130) that becomes the core issue for many of these individuals. Borrowing from the work of Lenore Terr (1991) and that of Solomon and Heide (1999), he suggested traumatic experiences be organized in terms of the consequences on human behavior into three basic categories: *Type I* refers to acute trauma that is normally the result of "a single overwhelming event that has not being preceded by other such event"; *Type II* refers to "long-standing exposure to persistent overwhelming events [or] 'existential' trauma"; and *Type III* refers to a much more extreme experience that "results from multiple and pervasive violent events beginning at an early age and continuing for years" (p. 117). Garbarino (2015) found that "emotional numbness, foreshortened sense of the future, rage, affective dysregulation, narcissism, impulsivity and dissociative symptoms" were prevalent in the people interviewed (p. 117). He also pointed out that memory retrieval is differentially experienced by these individuals, where those whose experience of trauma is categorized as Types I and II, memories of the traumatic events remain more accessible and thus more likely to be recognized and addressed in treatment. In the case of those for whom Type III applies, the memories of the traumatic events are less available for retrieval due to the disassociation and emotional detachment normally present. For these latter individuals, we are not referring to the operation of the normal repressive process described by Freud (1894/1896) in his theory of symptom formations for neurotic symptomatology, but rather a much more dissociative process is at play. This association gives rise to their inability to remember and provide a full and detailed account of the traumatic experience. Such a dissociation has major implications for diagnosis and treatment, with misdiagnoses becoming ever more likely.

There is another major consideration in this regard when examining people of color from minority communities that may further complicate the clinical picture, specially when involved with the criminal system. For many of these individuals their involvement with the legal system may be complicated by a perception of injustice due to the color of their skins, and where the antisocial behavior ascribed to them may be construed as a function of explicit and implicit biases and the systemic discrimination in the legal system frequently experienced by people of color. The extensive work with Black boys and adolescents described by Vaughans and Spielberg (2014) in their two edited volumes will provide the readers with a painful reminder of the various obstacles and trauma people of color have to contend with related to racism, discrimination, and blatant microaggression that make the attainment of their educational and professional goals a lot more challenging. This same issue was also amply addressed by Tummala-Narra (2021) in her recent book *Trauma and Racial Minority Immigrants*, but now focusing on immigrant populations.

Other findings suggest that we need to consider the involvement of some neurological abnormalities in those engaged in criminal behaviors. This seems to be more likely in the case of primary psychopaths, as abnormalities can be related to the findings of under-arousal, minimal anxiety, and difficulty making meaningful connections or problems with attachment found in these individuals (Meloy, 2002). The fact that habitual criminals are "chronically cortically underaroused" (Raine, 1993, as cited by Meloy & Shiva, 2007) or exhibit "reduced autonomic arousal in response to distress cues of others" (Pfabigan et al., 2014, p. 42) highlights the underline neurological-based deficits found in this group. An important finding in this regard is that "higher psychopathic-trait offenders were able to provide self-report in a way that let them appear to be as empathic" as those in the control groups—and thus "enabling them to know, yet not to feel, what others feel" (Pfabigan et al., 2014, p. 42); this finding may explain the glibness and superficial charm often found among this group (Huss, 2014). The extent to which these neurological abnormalities may have a hereditary basis was also raised by Meloy and Shiva (2007) in their analyses of findings with children and adolescents who were found to have callous-unemotional traits; proneness to thrill-seeking and fearlessness; deficits in responding to negative stimuli; who habituate more easily to distress in others; and who demonstrate lower autonomic reactivity to negative emotional stimuli. Such findings, particularly regarding their level of callousness led them to conclude that "heritability of these 'callous-unemotional' traits appears to be substantial" (p. 337).

From a more psychoanalytic perspective, Yakeley and Meloy (2012) and Meloy and Shiva (2007) also highlighted several insightful dynamics that may be at play with psychopaths and whose origin may be found very early in their developmental trajectory. According to these authors, psychopaths tend to show "a failure of internalization" where the normal process of incorporation becomes compromised by stress. Considering that this early form of internalization is first shown in the child's tendency to take and experience everything through its mouth, the nature of its immediate environment (e.g., hostile, abusive, depriving) becomes extremely important in providing the necessary guide to the development of basic trust in its environment (an issue amply addressed by Erikson, 1950/1963; Winnicott, 1965). They believe that this process can become contaminated by unpredictability and frustration of their basic needs due to failure during the early environment by parental figures (objects) who are responsible for administering care to the child. For these authors, these incorporative failures predicted subsequent problems with two kinds of internalizations: "identifications and introjections" in psychopathy. They see these identifications as serving a very important role, during the operation of which "the self or behavior are modified to increase resemblance to the object" (Meloy & Shiva, 2007, p. 339). Such a resemblance is expected to increase and solidify the opportunity for the development of meaningful bonding of the child with their parental figures, which once internalized becomes the foundation for superego-based morality (Freud, 1923). This process leads to the development of attachments

(Bowlby, 1969), considered by Fonagy (2004) as the necessary conditions for the development of the self with the ability to mentalize itself in reference to others and others in reference to itself. It is this quality that Fonagy (cited by Meloy & Shiva, 2007) found absent and considered a risk factor for violent criminality.

According to Fonagy (2004), this problem with mentation has a major implication for criminality as such a development is related to chronic problems with emotional detachment (or pathologies of attachment) that Bowlby (1944, 1969) found in many of the juvenile criminals he examined; Meloy and Shiva (2007) see this problem with attachment as resulting in apathy, self-absorption, preoccupation with nonhuman objects, no displays of emotion, tendency to be dismissive of others, and emotionally disorganized, all caused by constant maternal rejection and absence; it is caused also by the absence of meaningful involvement with a father figure, ultimately resulting in a failure, lack of internalization of the father's representation, or an "internal representation of the father that remains primitive" (p. 11), a point also made earlier by Fonagy and Target (1995).

Summarizing the work of Bowlby (1944, 1969), Winnicott (1971), Fonagy and Target (1995), Glasser (1978, 1998), Glover (1960), Hyatt-Williams (1998), and others, Yakeley and Meloy (2012) emphasized that the mind develops the capacity for representation or mentalization as the "key to human development and social interaction" (p. 3). They suggest that it is this capacity that becomes compromised in some personality disorders and violent individuals due to "environmental trauma and the disruptions to the attachment system, as well as constitutional factors" that tend to interfere with the normal developmental process. Once that process is interfered with and the normal development is derailed, it compromises "the capacity for mentalization" and leads to "the predominance of more primitive modes of subjective experience and psychological defenses" (p. 3); here they refer to defenses such as splitting and projective identification, which reflects a serious problem with self-cohesiveness. In some instances, it results in actual violence toward others. In this regard, they made references to a kind of violence that is meaningless and devoid of all symbolism where there is just "a visceral excitement or somatic gratification" (p. 5), as depicted in the movie *Silence of the Lambs* and likely to be present in the recent case of Aiden Fucci discussed earlier. The cases of Jeffrey Dahmer, Albert Fish, Tsutomu Miyazaki, and Armin Meiwes are also other possible examples in the same category (Javier et al., 2020a, 2020b).

For Glover (1960, as cited by Yakeley & Meloy, 2012), there is an intimate link to hate and anxiety in criminality, which becomes activated by frustration and other psychic changes, and that results in criminal behavior. In this context, the author contends that "both constitutional and environmental factors, including 'traumatic stimulation' and 'broken home'" (p. 6) should be considered to be at play. In the end, these authors suggest that we need to consider the different dynamics involved in the display of aggression with a primary source (or primary aggression) and aggression that is more reactive (or reactive aggression); for these authors, the latter should be seen as a function of a "more temporary 'functional' aggressive reactions to anxiety,'" and the former as a function of "a more permanent structural modification of the ego and superego by mechanisms such as unconscious identification with the aggressor . . . that could result in psychopathy" (p. 6).

Following a post-Kleinian, the authors also suggested another dynamic that could be at play in criminality; that is, the likelihood that individuals prone to violence to be dominated by persecutory anxieties they are unable to tolerate and that "they attempt to expel via projective identification" (p. 6). In that context, criminal acts are to be seen as "encapsulated unmetabolized death experiences . . . which overwhelms the mind and have to be completely projected in homicide or introjected in suicide" (p. 6), all representing the collapse of the capacity for symbolic thinking. For Winnicott (1986, 1988), however, who comes from the perspective that object relatedness supersedes aggression as an instinctual drive and that the individual is primarily interested in the object (or primarily object seeker), aggressive acts should be viewed within a much more sympathetic perspective to be construed as "the tendencies of anger, resentment, and violence as an attempt to regain the lost object" (Yakeley & Meloy, 2012, p. 7).

We recognize, however, that there is a lot more to the picture in the case of individuals whose criminal behaviors are categorized as "primary psychopathy" and thus the view of Glasser of violence as coming from two different sources may shed some additional light to these kinds of psychopathic behavior. For Glasser (1978, 1998), who also considers the genesis of aggression as resulting from the earlier maternal bond, a criminal act is guided by the need for self-preservation (or what Glasser refers to as "self-preservative violence"), and a violent act should be "considered a primitive response triggered by any threat to the physical or psychological self" (Yakeley & Meloy, 2012, p. 8). Such an attack may come from external sources on the person's self-esteem (related to experience of frustration, humiliation or insult to an ideal to what the person is attached) or coming from the personal psychic organization (or from "a sadistic superego, or fearing a loss of identity by feeling of disintegration and internal confusion") (Yakeley & Meloy, 2012, p. 8). We wonder if some of that dynamic may be operating in the case of Lori Vallow, referred to earlier in this chapter. We also see that in operation in criminal behaviors in reaction to a defendant's feeling "of being disrespected" by the target of the resulting violent assault. For Glasser (1978, 1998), such violent acts are "fundamental, immediate, and aimed at eliminating the source of danger"; it may also include "an attack on the person's own body," resulting in "self-harm or suicide" (p. 8). In other types of violence with a more sadomasochistic quality, the object of the attack "must be seen to suffer . . . [but] it must be preserved rather than eliminated" (Yakeley & Meloy, 2012, p. 8), with the act itself involving pleasure with no anxiety present.

Concluding Thoughts

In this chapter we highlighted the importance of distinguishing criminal behaviors for which we cannot find clear antecedents and explanations in early developmental history, from criminal behavior for which we can identify early trauma experienced during critical developmental period preceding the development and expression of aggressive and destructive behaviors. For this latter group of criminal behaviors, we provided extensive psychological and psychoanalytic explanations that may help contextualize the conditions more likely to trigger violent outbursts in these individuals, leading to criminal behaviors. For the former, a much more hereditary and neurological explanation seems to fit better to the cruelty, viciousness, callousness, and meticulousness of the planning in some of the most hideous crimes. Part of our fascination with criminal behaviors in general is because such behaviors go counter to our expectation of respect, propriety, and safety in our relationship with others.

In the end, we will be in the best position to decipher and understand the diverse expressions of criminal behaviors if we were to focus our attention on several core issues that have been found to underline criminal behaviors. In that context, when assessing and treating individuals with a history of criminal behaviors, we should consider focusing on the following, in addition to the standard forensic issues amply described by Huss (2014):

- Possible role of loss and trauma in the person's behavior
- Nature of the disruptions in the development of attachment or the inherited deficiencies in attachment capacity
- Nature and quality of the internal object world (including the relationship with the maternal and the paternal objects, and the self)
- Nature and quality of the superego development or the capacy to feel remorse
- Capacity for representation, symbolization, and mentalization
- Role of unconscious fantasy
- Role of conscious fantasy
- Development and capacity affecting self-regulation.
- Development and limitations of the ego defenses, particularly the predominant use of more primitive defenses (e.g., devaluation, denial, projection, and projective identification)
- Nature and quality of reality testing or the ability to distinguish between fantasy and external reality
- Recognition of the neurobiological underpinnings of all violent acts

The best treatment intervention then should also recognize the severe psychopathology normally present in violent criminals and thus the importance of limiting our expectations of how much change we can expect. Yakeley and Meloy (2012) suggest that if we were to foster "the development of a psychic function in the patient's mind that can begin to experience and tolerate loss, remorse, concern, and empathy" we would have accomplished a monumental step in helping these patients "replace action modes of thinking and relating" (p. 21). In this case, a replacement for one that is more likely to foster respectful relatedness with other, with the understanding that there will be moments of regression and reenactment along the way. They also suggest considering pharmacological intervention as an option to help these patients contain and control their affect. We add that any intervention that works systematically on realigning and reprograming (or rewiring) the way personal scripts/schemas are automatically deployed as criminal and violent acts (as amply delineated by Warburton & Anderson, 2018), will go a long way in helping those interested in changing the ways they relate with themselves and others to then be characterized by respectful mutuality.

The challenge for all of us, however, is how are we to recognize and contextualize in our assessment of criminal acts perpetuated by individuals whose criminal histories may have been preceded by serious, continuous, and debilitating traumas experiences related to racism, prejudices, discrimination, and various kinds of systemic aggressions and microaggressions. We must do so without, in the process, being construed directly or indirectly as endorsing that such an act was justified because of the systemic injustice they may have experienced. Our effort here is only in keeping with the *Jurisprudence* principle, to provide the necessary information on the possible factors and dynamics that may have been at play and that may be helpful for the court and the legal system to know in the adjudication of justice. In the end, it is also meant to encourage the court to consider including possible psychological interventions in its decision during the period of incarceration and beyond.

10

Summary and Conclusions

The primary goal of this book is to promote the use of integrated psychotherapy as the most effective mental health delivery system. We begin by describing current mental health treatment, then indicating the clinical value of psychoanalysis, the growth of pluralism, specific clinical examples of the integrated approach, and the variable path of effective integration. We also include a review of outcome research with its numerous problems and exceptions, discuss the role of language in the therapeutic exchange, consider possible neuroscientific contributions to the dialogue, and then show a specific application, understanding criminal behavior. Now we are at the point of summarizing our support and drawing conclusions.

Our concept of integration involves dividing psychotherapies broadly into "outer-life" and "inner-life" focused approaches and integrating their aims in the varying procedures based on the needs of individual patients. We begin with the current type of help that is provided by a singular behavioral approach, which includes all the variants focused on altering behavior, such as trauma, specific symptoms, and includes medications. These are "outer-life" therapies aimed at changing how a person acts, with the possibility that behavioral changes will also be accompanied by thought and emotional changes.

In contrast, there are "inner-life" therapies that focus on feeling and accompanying thinking with the possibility that behavioral change will also occur that is reflective of the internal exploration. Thinking and feeling are involved in both approaches, but there is also a distinctive difference in emphasis that supports our categorization. For example, it is possible to alter racist behavior without changing racist thoughts and feelings. Our point in drawing the distinction is to highlight the therapeutic aim of the different approaches, thought always being involved to some degree in any talk therapy, and medication involves thoughtful purpose by the providers. Even action could be construed as implied thought, but is not necessarily congruent with actual thought, nor with emotional states.

For behavior therapies success is measured by behavior change. For example, in the case of anger management, improvement means a patient shows less anger. However, that change does not automatically mean the person feels less angry or has less angry thoughts. At the same time, there is hope that showing less anger means also feeling and thinking less anger. That logic is more wish than proven reality.

In inner-life therapies hope is also apparent in that the emphasis is on self-exploration to understand feelings and the way that one thinks regarding the feelings, with the wish that logic will dictate behavior change as well. The emphasis is on self-understanding with the belief that self-knowledge will logically result in altered behavior, but again, this is a wish. Inner-life therapies give limited attention to symptom removal, focusing more on developmental factors, while outer-life therapies see limited value in that type of exploration. The why of behavior is of great significance, while behavior therapists emphasize new behavior.

In both types of therapies, there is what could be termed total success, meaning that everything changed, though each has accepted the more limited goal as curative. As a result, most of the time it is a split decision, meaning the person acts different but feels the same, or feels different but acts the same, so not congruent, but in turn, not that impressive. For us, this adds up to the probability that if time were taken to tend to it all, behavior, thoughts, and feelings, the results would be more impressive.

It would be helpful if we had improvement data to back up our assertion, but mental health treatment has a history of looking for the "cure" in a singular fashion of reflecting a relatively narrow goal and assuming, really wishing, for an entire alteration of the mental illness. In modern times, first, it was psychoanalysis, which did not really make the effort to demonstrate its effectiveness while over-promising what it could and would do. The revolutionary impact of its conceptualizations passed, the treatment foundered, there was a lack of desired effectiveness, it was lengthy and costly, and it got usurped by a behavioral tide of brevity, cost-effective estimates that fit nicely with managed care, and supposed evidence of behavioral change. Now we are within this behavioral wave, which turns out not to be that effective either, and damaging in unintended ways, such as the drastic reduction in long-term mental health facilities and the system of revolving door treatments in service of economic goals.

In our chapter on treatment effectiveness, we have pointed out the obstacles to producing reliable and valid indices of improvement. This is an area of complexity that so far does not have a viable solution. At best we can conclude that all psychotherapies are effective to some degree, but that psychotherapy needs to be customized to the patient, with the understanding that there are structural variables that are personalized and difficult to factor into outcomes. At this point, we can state that no one therapeutic approach is consistently effective, but in general, psychotherapy is helpful, and in some instances, significantly effective. We believe that this supports our conclusion that integrative therapy is likely to be the most effective approach.

Based on our observations of current psychotherapists we sense there is movement in that direction, and we have cited authors who describe their work that way. Within the psychoanalytic community, which is our area of familiarity, there has been a remarkable growth of pluralism and a willingness to move away from orthodoxy and to retrofit concepts and techniques, but not yet a stated willingness to embrace an integrated model. We believe it is likely that behavioral approaches will also reflect expansion and differentials of emphasis, though we do not consider ourselves qualified enough to suggest specifics beyond that the inner-life requires more consideration. There is indeed something to be said for the examined mind as a component of behavioral change.

Since psychoanalysis is the current outlier and needs elevation to be a significant factor in integrative treatment, we include the following quote: "As someone who has suffered with depression and has a family history of depression and suicide, I consider myself fortunate to have found two psychoanalysts who are willing and able to sit with me beside the abyss before it swallowed me whole. Their presence and constancy enabled some daylight eventually to sneak through" (Anderson, 2023, p. 15).

We are living in a time of increasing uncertainty and complexity. The world appears to be getting more difficult to understand and navigate. The apprehension greeting the advances of artificial intelligence is indicative of the wonder as to what lies ahead of us. The *Wall Street Journal* repeatedly prints sections on the Future of Everything. Mental health is likely to be more of an issue than it has already been during COVID.

Integrated psychotherapy is an appropriate next step, but for treatment to be effective we need to have a better environment than our present delivery system. When Bernie Sanders advocates Medicare for all he is conceptually on target for supporting the right to mental health. Funding underlies the issue of effectiveness. Our health system is currently constructed so that the availability of mental services rests upon the discretion of insurers for most of the population. This mitigates the motivation for provision from expressed needs by patients and providers because the gatekeepers have an economic incentive to keep services restricted based on economic factors. For mental health such an incentive is to use "evidence-based" therapies that are duration- and cost-limited. The use of "evidence" appears reasonable, except with mental disorders, as we have demonstrated, the "evidence" is less than valid or reliable. Furthermore, the composition of both mental disorders and their therapies limits the possible confidence in using effectiveness studies to determine psychotherapy duration and cost. A patient's need and provider's opinion are more accurate measures. There is no evidence of runaway costs before the introduction of managed care, and given patient ambivalence about seeking help and being in therapy, excessive cost is unlikely.

For psychotherapy to be effective over a life span, which is particularly desirable for the development and maintenance of a healthy and productive society, mental illness has to be understood as a potentially chronic hazard with episodes and varying degrees of severity. With all the violence that appears to be taking place the control factor is not going to rest on gun control alone, but this needs to be accompanied by an awareness of the necessity for understanding the propensity of people to be violent and an exploration of their reasons for taking such action. Mitigating violence is very much a mental health issue, as is coping with unemployment or dealing with a pandemic. We need better mental health; people have a right to it and there is a need for more adequate funding.

Medicare has the potential for being a workable funding model, although, regarding mental health it is cost-conscious in a disappointing way. For example, there has been a year-by-year reduction in amounts allowed for psychotherapy and there is pressure to use the most time-restrictive codes (less cost) therapy codes. We are aware of the limitations that seem inherent in a bureaucracy, but modifications are to be expected. The thrust should be to make psychotherapy available to whoever needs it whenever it is needed, with patients having the right to expect it. Given that indeed it is often difficult to get people to seek therapy, and then to have them stay with it long enough for it to be helpful, we reiterate that the cost of such availability should be unlimited because it is going to be a rather small fraction of a total health care budget. Also, decisions about procedure and duration need to be made by the patient-therapist combination, not by an employee of the funding entity, and integrated procedures should be available. We need to find what works and then do what works, instead of focusing on either a popular favorite or the cheapest model.

We understand that fiscal solvency for the government is an issue, and that the need for health care is a large item, but it is clear, that when it comes to a threat to the health of our society, cost is not allowed to be an obstacle. That has been evident during the pandemic. Nulia, a medical doctor writing in the *New York Times* in 2023, sees health insurers as a major problem in providing adequate health care, and suggests a single-payer plan as the best solution. Dean and Talbot (2023), medical doctors, see the current system as doing moral harm to providers. The current approach tends to combine socialism and capitalism in a way that maximizes the problems of each, arbitrariness and profit.

Our focus is on only one part of the system, mental health, which we feel is unfairly targeted for cost reductions because of the limits involved in measuring its efficacy. We certainly wish it could be reliably and validly measured as to treatment effectiveness due to difficulties in controlling the many factors normally involved in the therapeutic transaction, as extensively discussed in Chapter 6 earlier; what can be measured, and is continually apparent, is the detrimental effects of mental illness. They represent the most powerful incentive for unlimited care, and that cost is marginal compared to other health problems. For example, the treatment of schizophrenia, potentially a lengthy process with often, at best, palliative results, is still relatively inexpensive compared to cancer care. Of course, mental illness is rarely fatal, yet rarely curable, just persistent. Unfortunately, it is the type of illness that becomes an easy target for cost reduction, multiple elements at work, namely uncertain duration, uncertain outcome, so an obvious avenue for cost control that can be made to appear reasonable. Also, adding to the cost and session limits, are the networks that limit patient access to providers of their choice. There is no evidence to support the value of these restrictions to patients, yet they remain in place and are barriers to psychotherapeutic effectiveness as well. We believe the chronicity and extent of mental illness is very sufficient evidence to support unrestricted access to therapeutic services, and these services should involve integrative psychotherapy for maximal effectiveness.

References

Ablon, J. S., & Jones, E. S. (2005). On analytic process. *Journal of the American Psychoanalytic Association, 53*, 541–568.

Ainsworth, M. D., Blehar, M. C., Waters, E., & Wall, S. (1978). *Patterns of attachment: A psychological study of the strange situation.* Erlbaum.

Allen, J. G., & Fonagy, P. (2017). Trauma. In P. Luyten, L. C. Mayes, P. Fonagy, M. Target, & S. J. Blatt, *Handbook of psychodynamic approaches to psychopathology* (pp. 165–198). Guilford Press.

Almajera, A. (2022, December 7). I'm a witness to a mental health crisis. *New York Times.* https://www.nytimes.com/2022/12/07/opinion/nyc-paramedic-mental-health-crisis.html

Anderson, J. (2023). Letters to the editor. *New York Times.*

Aron, L., & Starr, K. (2013). *A psychotherapy for the people: Toward a progressive psychoanalysis.* Routledge.

Auchincloss, E. L., & Samberg, E. (Eds.) (2012). *Psychoanalytic terms and concepts.* Yale University Press.

Axelrod, S. D., Naso, R.C., & Rosenberg, L. M. (Eds.) (2018). *Progress in psychoanalysis: Envisioning the future of the profession.* Routledge.

Bachrach, H. M., & Leaff, L. A. (1978). "Analyzability": A systemic review of the clinical and quantitative literature. *Journal of the American Psychoanalytic Association, 26*(4), 881–920. https://doi.org/10.1177/000306517802600409

Bakhshani, N. (2014). Impulsivity: A predisposition toward risky behaviors. *International Journal of High Risk Behaviors and Addiction, 3*(2), e20428. doi: 10.5812/ijhrba.20428

Barlow, D. H. (Ed.) (2008). *Clinical handbook of psychological disorders: A step-by-step treatment manual* (4th ed.). Guilford Press.

Barsness, P. E. (2021). Therapeutic practices in relational psychoanalysis: A qualitative study. *Psychoanalytic Psychology, 38*, 22–30.

Beidel, D., & Frueh, B. C. (Eds.) (2018). *Adult psychopathology and diagnosis.* Wiley.

Bellak, L., & Goldsmith, L. A. (Eds.) (1984). *The broad scope of ego function assessment.* John Wiley.

Bellak, L., & Meyers, B. (1975). Ego function assessment and analyzability. *International Journal of Psychoanalysis, 2*, 415–427.

Bendezú, J. J., Loughlin-Presnal, J. E., & Wadsworth, M. E. (2019). Attachment security moderates effects of uncontrollable stress on preadolescent Hypothalamic-Pituitary-Adrenal Axis Responses: Evidence of regulatory fit. *Psychological Science, 7*(6), 1355–1371.

Benjamin, J. (2018). *Beyond doer and done to: Recognition theory, intersubjectivity and the third.* Routledge.

Bialystok, E. (2001). *Bilingualism in development: Language, literacy, and cognition.* Cambridge University Press.

Bialystok, E., & Cummins, J. (2000). Language, cognition, and education of bilingual children. In E. Bialystok (Ed.), *Language processing in bilingual children* (pp. 222–232). Cambridge University Press.

Blagys, M. D., & Hlisenroth, M. J. (2000). Distinctive features of short-term psychodynamic-Interpersonal psychotherapy. A review of the psychotherapy process literature. *Clinical Psychology: Science and Practice, 7*, 167–188.

Bowlby, J. (1969). *Attachment and loss: Attachment* (Vol. 1). Basic Books.

Bowlby, J. (1988). *A secure base: Clinical applications of attachment theory*. Routledge.

Bowlby, S. J. (1944). Forty-four juvenile thieves: Their characters and home life. *International Journal of Psychoanalysis, 25*(19–52), 107–127.

Bryant, R. A., & Datta, S. (2019). Reconsolidating intrusive distressing memories by thinking attachment figures: Brief report. *Clinical Psychological Science, 7*(6), 1249–1256. doi:10.1177/2167702619866387

Bucci, W. (2021). Overview of the referential process: The operation of language within and between people. *Journal of Psycholinguist Research, 50*, 3–15. https://doi.org/10.1007/s10936-021-09759-2

Buechler, S. (2019). *Psychoanalytic approaches to problems in living*. Routledge.

Bulhan, H. A. (1985). *Frantz Fanon and the psychology of oppression*. Plenum.

Burgess, K. B., Marshall, P. J., Rubin, K. H., & Fox, N. A. (2003). Infant attachment and temperament as predictors of subsequent externalizing problems and cardiac physiology. *Journal of Child Psychopathology and Psychiatry, 44*, 819–831.

Busch, F. (2014). *Creating a psychoanalytic mind*. Routledge.

Busch, F. N. (2018). *Psychodynamic approaches to behavioral change*. American Psychiatric Publishing.

Buxbaum, E. (1949). The role of a second language in the formation of ego and superego. *International Journal of Psychiatry, 18*, 279–289.

Chapman, L. K., DeLapp, R. C. T., & Williams, M. T. (2018). Impact of race, ethnicity and culture on the expression and assessment of psychopathology. In D. C. Beidel & B. C. Frueh (Eds.), *Adult psychopathology and diagnosis* (8th ed., pp. 131–156). Wiley.

Cherry, S., Aizaga, K. H., & Roose, S. P. (2009). The Columbia longitudinal study of postgraduate career development and analytic practice; Four years of experience. *Journal of the American Psychoanalytic Association, 57*, 196–199.

Clarkin, J. F., Fonagy, P., Levy, K. N., & Bateman, A. (2017). Borderline personality disorder. In P. Luyten, L. C. Mayes, P. Fonagy, M. Target, & S. J. Blatt (Eds.). *Handbook of psychodynamic approaches to psychopathology* (pp. 353–380). Guilford Press.

Clauss-Ehlers, C. S. Millan, F., & Zhao, C. J. (2018). Understanding domestic violence within the Latino-Hispanic/Latinx context: Environmental, culturally relevant assessment tool. In R. A. Javier & W. G. Herron (Eds.). *Understanding domestic violence: Theories, challenges, and remedies* (pp. 237–262). Rowman & Littlefield.

Cleckley, H. (1941). *The mask of sanity*. Mosby.

Colli, A., Gagliardini, G., Guerrini Degl'Innocenti, B. D., Ponsi, M., Rossi Monti, M., & Foresti, G. (2020). What psychoanalysts do in their everyday clinical practice: Empirically derived prototypes of the psychoanalytic process. *Psychoanalytic Psychotherapy, 37*, 136–147.

Collins, A. M., & Loftus, E. F. (1975). A spreading activation theory of semantic processing. *Psychological Review, 82*, 407–428.

Comas-Diaz, L., & Jacobsen, F. M. (1991). Ethnocultural transference and countertransference in the therapeutic dyad. *American Journal of Orthopsychiatry, 61*(3), 392–402. https://doi.org/10.1037/h0079267.

CourtTV (2023, March 21). Aiden Fucci Sentencing Hearing: Powerful Victim ... - Court TV. www.courttv.com. Retrieved July 28, 2023.

Courtois, C. A., & Ford, J. (Eds.) (2009). *Treating complex traumatic stress disorders: An evidence-based guide*. Guilford Press.

Cramer. P. (2006). *Protecting the self: Defense mechanisms in action*. Guilford Press.

Cramer, P. (2008). Seven pillars of defense theory. *Social and Personality Psychology Compass, 2*, 1963–1981.

Crecci, M. B. (2010). Roundtable discussion: What are we learning from the division's practice survey? *Psychologist-Psychoanalyst, 30*, 14.

Cuijpers, P., Cristea, I. A., Karyotaki, E., Reijnders, M., & Huibers, M. J. (2016). How effective are cognitive behavior therapies for major depression and anxiety disorders? A meta-analytic update of the evidence. *World Psychiatry, 15*, 245–258.

Cuijpers, P., Karyotaki, E., Reijnders. M., & Ebert, D. D. (2018). Was Eysenck right after all? A reassessment of the effects of psychotherapy for adult depression. *Epidemiology and Psychiatric Sciences*. https://doi.org/10.1017/ S2045796018000057

Cuijpers, P., Reijnders, M., & Huibers, M. J. H. (2019). The role of common factors in psychotherapy outcome. *Annual Review of Clinical Psychology, 15*, 207–231. https://doi.org/10.1146/annurev-clinpsy-050718-095424

Cuijpers P, van Straten, A., Bohlmeijer E., Hollon, S. D., & Andersson, G. (2010). The effects of psychotherapy for adult depression are overestimated: a meta-analysis of study quality and effect size. *Psychological Medicine, 40*, 211–223.

Dana, R. H. (1993). *Multicultural assessment perspectives for professional psychology*. Allyn & Bacon.

Dean, W., & Talbot, S. (2023). *If I betray these words*. Stueforth.

Demos, E. V. (1998). Differentiating the repetition compulsion from trauma through the lens of Tompkins's script theory: A response to Russell. In J. G. Teicholz & D. Kriegman (Eds.), *Trauma, repetition compulsion, and affect regulation: The work of Paul Russell* (pp. 67–104). Other Press.

Downing, D. L., & Mills, J. (Eds.). (2017). *Outpatient treatment of psychosis. Psychodynamic approaches to evidence-based practice*. Routledge.

Eagle, M. (2022). *Toward a unified psychoanalytic theory*. Routledge.

Eagle, M. N. (2011). *From clinical to contemporary psychoanalysis. A critique and integration*. Routledge.

Eagle, M. N. (2018a). *Core concepts in classical psychoanalysis*. Routledge.

Eagle, M. N. (2018b). *Core concepts in contemporary psychoanalysis*. Routledge.

El-Jamil, F. & Abi-Hashem, N. (2018). Family maltreatment and domestic violence among Arab Middle Easterners: A psychological, cultural, religious, and legal examination. In R. A. Javier & W. G. Herron (Eds.). *Understanding domestic violence: Theories, challenges, and remedies* (pp. 179–212). Rowman & Littlefield.

Elliott, R., Bohart, A. C., Watson, J. C., & Greenberg, L.S. (2011). Empathy. *Psychotherapy, 48*(1): 43–49.

Erikson, E. H. (1950/1963) *Childhood and Society*. New York: W.W. Norton & Company, Inc.

Etezady, M. H. (2018). Introduction. In M. H. Etezady, M. Blom, & M. Davis (Eds.), *Psychoanalytic trends in theory and practice: The second century of the talking cure*. Lexington Books.

Foa, E. B. (1997). Psychological processes related to recovery from a trauma and an effective treatment for PTSD. In R. Yehuda & A. C. McFarlane (Eds.), *Psychobiology of posttraumatic stress disorder* (pp. 410–424). New York Academy of Sciences.

Fonagy, P. (2004). Early life trauma and the psychogenesis and prevention of violence. *Annals of the New York Academy of Sciences, 1036*, 181–200.

Fonagy, P., & Luyten, P. (2009). A developmental, mentalization-based approach to the understanding and treatment of borderline personality disorder. *Development and Psychopathology, 21*, 1355–1381.

Fonagy, P., & Target, M. (1997). Attachment and reflective function: Their role in self-organization. *Development and Psychopathology, 9*, 679–700.

Fonagy, P., & Target, M. (1995). Understanding the violent patient: The use of the body and the role of the father. *International Journal of Psychoanalysis, 767*, 487–501.

Foster, R. (1996). Assessing the psychodynamic function of language in the bilingual patient. In R. Foster, M. Moskowitz, & R. A. Javier (Eds.), *Reaching across boundaries, culture and class: Widening the scope of psychotherapy* (pp. 243–263). Jason Aronson.

Freud, A. (1966). *The ego and the mechanisms of defense* (Revised ed.). International Universities Press. Originally published 1936.

Freud, A. (1973). *The ego and the mechanisms of defense*. Routledge.

Freud, S. (1894). The neuro-psychoses of defense. In J. Strachey (Trans.), *The standard edition of the complete psychological works of Sigmund Freud* (Vol. III, pp. 43–61). Hogarth Press.

Freud, S. (1896). Further remarks on the neuro-psychoses of defense. In J. Strachey (Trans.), *The standard edition of the complete psychological works of Sigmund Freud* (Vol. III, pp. 159–185). Hogarth Press.

Freud, S. (1905). Three essays on the theory of sexuality. *SE, 7*, 125–243.

Freud, S. (1914/1981). Remembering, repeating, and working through (Further recommendations on the technique of psychoanalysis II). In J. Strachey (Trans.), *The standard edition of the complete psychological works of Sigmund Freud* (Vol. 12, pp. 145–156). Hogarth Press.

Freud, S. (1915). Instincts and their vicissitudes. In J. Strachey (Trans.), *The standard edition of the complete psychological works of Sigmund Freud* (pp. 109–140). Hogarth Press

Freud, S. (1923). The ego and the id. In J. Strachey (Trans.), *The standard edition of the complete psychological works of Sigmund Freud* (Vol. XIX, pp. 3–66). Hogarth Press.

Freud, S. (1928). Dostoevsky and parricide. In J. Strachey (Trans.), *The standard edition of the complete psychological works of Sigmund Freud* (Vol. XXI). Hogarth Press.

Freud, S. (1937). Analysis terminable and interminable. In J. Strachey (Trans.), *The standard edition of the complete psychological works of Sigmund Freud* (Vol. 23, pp. 209–253). Hogarth Press.

Freud, S. (1913/1981). On the beginning of treatment (Further recommendations on the technique of psycho-analysis I). In J. Strachey (Trans.), *The standard edition of the complete psychological works of Sigmund Freud* (Vol. 12, pp. 123–144). Hogarth Press. (Original work published 1913.)

Furukawa, T. A., Noma, H., Caldwell, D. M., Honyashiki, M., & Shinohara, K., et al. (2014). Waiting list may be a nocebo condition in psychotherapy trials: a contribution from network meta-analysis. *Acta Psychiatrica Scandinavica, 130*, 181–192.

Garbarino, J. (2015). *Listening to killers: Lesson learned from my 20 years as a psychological expert witness in murder cases*. University of California Press.

Gardner, D. (2010, September). *Thomas Hobbes and Niccolo Machiavelli: A comparison.* Retrieved March 15, 2023, from https://www.e-ir.info/2010/09/01/thomas-hobbes-and-niccolo-machiavelli-a-comparison/

Gazzilo, F., Dazzi, N., DeLuca, E., Radonmonti, G., & Silberschatz, G. (2020). Attachment disorganization and severe psychopathology: A possible dialogue between attachment theory and control mastery theory. *Psychoanalytic Psychology, 37*, 173–184.

Gediman, H. K. (2011). Cutting edge controversies: True and false dichotomies. *Psychoanalytic Review, 98*, 613–632.

Gediman, H. K. (2018). *Building bridges. Selected psychoanalytic papers of Helen K. Gediman*. International Psychoanalytic Books.

Gherovici, P., & Christian, C. (Eds.) (2019). *Psychoanalysis in the barrios: Race, class, and the unconscious*. Routledge.

Gill, H. S. (1988). Working through resistances of intrapsychic and environmental origin [Case report]. *International Journal of Psychoanalysis, 69*(Pt 4), 535–550. PMID: 3220677

Glasser, M. (1978). The role of superego in exhibitionism. *International Journal of Psychoanalytic Psychology, 7,* 333–352.

Glasser, M. (1998). On violence: A preliminary communication. *International Journal of Psychoanalysis, 79,* 887–902.

Glover, F. (1960). *The roots of crime.* Imago Publishing.

Gnaulati, E. (2018). *Saving talk therapy.* Beacon Press.

Gold, S. D., Marx, B. P., Soler-Baillo, J. M., & Sloan, D. M. (2005). Is life stress more traumatic than traumatic stress? *Journal of Anxiety Disorders, 19,* 687–698.

Goldberg, S. H. (2022). Discussion of "from *what* to *how*: A conversation with Stefano Bolognini on emotional attunement" by Luca Nicoli and Stefao Bolognini. *Psychoanalytic Quarterly, 91*(3), 477–488. doi:10.1080/00332828.2022.2118503

Goldstein, E. B., & Cacciamani, L. (2022). *Sensation and perception.* Cengage Learning.

Gonzalez, A., Weersing, V. R., Warnick, E. M., Scahill, L. D., & Woolston, J. L. (2011). Predictors of treatment attrition among an outpatient clinic sample of youths with clinically significant anxiety. *Administration and Policy in Mental Health and Mental Health Services Research, 38*(5), 356–367.

Greenberg, J. R., & Mitchell, S. A. (1983). *Object relations in psychoanalytic theory.* Harvard University Press.

Greenson, R. (1950). The mother tongue and the mother. *International Journal of Psychoanalysis, 31,* 18–23.

Greenson, R. (1968). *The technique and practice of psychoanalysis* (Vol. I). International Universities Press.

Hare, R. D. (1996). Psychopathy: A clinical construct whose time has come. *Criminal Justice and Behavior, 23,* 23–54.

Hare, R. D. (2001). Psychopaths and their nature: Some implications for understanding human predator violence. In A. Raine & J. San Martin (Eds.), *Violence and psychopathy* (pp. 5–34). Academic/Plenum Publishers.

Hart, S. F., & Dempster, R. J. (1997). Impulsivity and psychopathy. In C. D. Webster & M. A. Jackson (Eds.). *Impulsivity: Theory, assessment, and treatment* (pp. 212–232). Guilford Press.

Hartmann, H. (1939/1958). *Ego psychology and the problem with adaptation.* International Universities Press.

Hartmann, H. (1958). *Essays on ego psychology: Selected problems in psychoanalytic theory.* International Universities Press.

Hayes, S. C., Follettte, V. M., & Linehan, M. M. (Eds.) (2004). *Mindfulness and acceptance: Expanding the cognitive-behavioral approaches.* Guilford Press.

Herron, W. G., & Javier, R. A. (2019). The impact of pluralism. *Psychology and Psychological Research International Journal, 4,* 1–9.

Hill, J., & Sharp, H. (2017). Conduct disorders. In P. Luyten, L. C. Mayes, P. Fonagy, M. Target, & S. J. Blatt (Eds.), *Handbook of psychodynamic approaches to* psychopathology (pp. 406–425). Guilford Press.

Holmes, D. E. (2006). The wrecking effects of race and social class on self and success. *The Psychoanalytic Quarterly, 75*(1), 215–235. doi:10.1002/ j.2167-4086.2006.tb00038.x

Huss, M. T. (2014). *Forensic Psychology: Research, clinical practice, and applications.* Wiley.

Hyatt-Williams, A. (1998). *Cruelty, violence, and murder: Understanding the criminal mind.* Jason Aronson.

Jaffe, L. (2014). *How talking cures. Revealing Freud's contributions to all psychotherapies.* Rowman & Littlefield.

Javier, R. A. (1995). Vicissitudes of autobiographical memories in bilingual analysis. *Psychoanalytic Psychology, 12,* 429–438.

Javier, R. A. (1996). In search of repressed memories in bilingual individuals. In R. M., Perez Foster, M. Moskowitz, & R. A. Javier (Eds.), *Reaching across boundaries of culture and class* (pp. 225–241). Jason Aronson.

Javier, R. A. (2007). *The bilingual mind: Thinking, feeling, and speaking in two languages.* Springer Science.

Javier, R. A., & Herron, W. G. (1992). Psychoanalysis, the Hispanic poor, and the disadvantage: Application and reconsideration. *Journal of the American Academy of Psychoanalysis, 20,* 455–476.

Javier, R. A., & Lamela, M. (2020). Cultural and linguistic issues in assessing trauma in a forensic context. In R. A. Javier, E. A. Owen, & J. A. Maddux (Eds.), *Assessing trauma in forensic contexts* (pp. 151–179). Springer Science.

Javier, R. A., & Owen, E. A. (2020). Trauma and its vicissitudes in forensic contexts: An introduction. In R. A. Javier, E. A. Owen, & J. A. Maddux (Eds), *Assessing trauma in forensic contexts* (pp. 1–34). Springer.

Javier, R. A., & Yussef, M. B. (1998). A Latino perspective on the role of ethnicity in the development of moral values: Implications for psychoanalytic theory and practice. In R. A. Javier & W. G. Herron (Eds.), *Personality development and psychotherapy in our diverse society: A source book.* Jason Aronson.

Javier, R. A., Owen, E. A., & Maddux, J. A. (2020a). Trauma and its trajectory in criminal behaviors: Case studies exercise assignments. In R. A., Javier, E. A. Owen, & J. A. Maddux (Eds). *Assessing trauma in forensic contexts* (pp. 509–646). Springer.

Javier, R. A., Owen, E. A., &. Maddux, J. A (Eds.) (2020b). *Assessing trauma in forensic contexts.* Springer.

Jessberger, S., & Gage, F. H. (2008). Stem-cell-associated structural and functional plasticity in the aging Hippocampus. *Psychology and Aging, 23,* 684–691. doi: 10.1037/a0014188

Jurist, E. L. (2010). Eliot Jurist interviews Peter Fonagy. *Psychoanalytic Psychology, 1,* 2–7.

Jurist, E. L. (2018). A defense of strong pluralism in psychoanalysis. Mentalizing the hermeneutic-science debate. In S. D. Axelrod, R. C. Naso, & L. M. Rosenberg (Eds.), *Progressive psychoanalysis: Envisioning the future of the profession* (pp. 17–35). Routledge.

Kadzin, A. E. (2007). Mediators and mechanisms of change in psychotherapy research. *Annual Review of Clinical Psychology, 3,* 1–27.

Kadzin, A. E., Stolar, M. J., & Marciano, P. L. (1995). Risk factors for dropping out of treatment among White and Black families. *Journal of Family Psychology, 9*(4), 402–417. https://doi.org/10.1037/0893-3200.9.4.402

Kernberg, O. (1984). *Severe personality disorders.* Yale University Press.

Kernberg, O. F. (2019). Therapeutic implications of transference structures in various personality pathologies. *Journal of the American Psychoanalytic Association, 67,* 951–986.

Kernberg, O. F., Yeomans, F. E., Clarkin, J. F., & Levy, K. N. (2008). Transference-focused psychotherapy: Overview and update. *International Journal of Psychoanalysis, 89,* 601–620.

Koestler, F. A. (2004). *The unseen minority: A social history of blindness in the United States.* AFB Press.

Lafarge, L. (2022). Three papers on the concept of neutrality: Editor's introduction. Lambert, M. J. (1992). Psychotherapy outcome research: implications for integrative and eclectical therapists, In J. C. Norcross & Goldfield, M. R. (Eds), *Handbook of Psychotherapy Integration* (pp. 94–129). Basic Books.

Landin-Romero, R., Moreno-Alcazar, A., Pagani, M., & Amann, B. L. (2018). How does eye movement desensitization and reprocessing therapy work? A systematic review on suggested mechanisms of action. *Frontiers in Psychology, 9,* 1395. doi: 10.3389/fpsyg.2018.01395

Leidenfrost, C. M., & Antonius, D. (2020). Incarceration and trauma: A challenge for the mental health care delivery system. In R. A. Javier, E. A. Owen, & J. A. Maddux (Eds). *Assessing trauma in forensic contexts* (pp. 85–150). Springer.

Levenson, H. (2010). *Brief dynamic therapy.* American Psychological Association.

Lichtenberg, J. D. (1989). *Psychoanalysis and motivation.* Analytic Press.

Lichtenstein, D. (2018). Multiplicity and rigor in psychoanalysis. In S. D. Axelrod, R. C. Naso, & L. M. Rosenberg (Eds.), *Progress in psychoanalysis. Envisioning the future of the profession* (pp. 78–97). Routledge.

Lingardi, V., & McWilliams, N. (Eds.) (2017). *Psychodynamic diagnostic manual* (2nd ed.). Guilford Press.

Luria, A. (1973). *The working brain: An introduction to neuropsychology.* Basic Books.

Luria, A. (1981). *Language and cognition.* Winston.

Luria, A., & Yudovich, F. (1968). *Speech and the development of the mental processes in the child.* Staples Press.

Luyten, P., & Blatt, S. J. (2017). The psychodynamic approach to diagnosis and classification. In P. Luyten, L. C. Mayes, P. Fonagy, M. Target, & S. J. Blatt (Eds.). *Handbook of psychodynamic approaches to psychopathology* (pp. 87–109). Guilford Press.

Luyten, P., Mayes, L. C., Fonagy, P., Target, M., & Blatt, S. J. (2017). *Handbook of psychodynamic approaches to psychopathology.* Guilford Press.

Mahlberg, N. T. (2018). Looking back while moving forward: Integrating developmental psychoanalysis and contemporary clinical practice. In S. D. Axelrod, R. C. Naso, and L. M. Rosenberg (Eds.), *Progress in Psychoanalysis. Envisioning the future of the profession* (pp. 199–218). Routledge.

Mahler, M. S. (1979a). *Selected papers of Margaret S. Mahler: Infantile psychosis and early contribution* (Vol. 1). Jason Aronson.

Mahler, M. S. (1979b). *Selected papers of Margaret S. Mahler: Separation-individuation* (Vol. II). Jason Aronson.

Mahler, M. S., Pine, F., & Bergman, A. (1975). *The psychological birth of the human infant-symbiosis and individuation.* Basic Books.

Makari, G. (2008). *Revolution in the mind: The creation of psychoanalysis.* HarperCollins.

Marcos, L. R. (1976). Linguistic dimensions in the bilingual patient. *American Journal of Psychoanalysis, 36,* 347–354.

McClanahan, B., & South, N. (2020). 'All knowledge begins with the senses': Towards a sensory criminology. *British Journal of Criminology, 60*(1), 3–23. https://doi.org/10.1093/bjc/azz052

McClendon, J., Dean, K. E. & Galovski, T. (2020) Addressing diversity in PTSD treatment: Disparities in treatment engagement and outcome among patients of color. *Current Treatment Options in Psychiatry, 7,* 275–290.

McCormick, A. (1950). The prison's role in crime prevention. *Journal of Criminal Law & Criminology, 41,* 36–48.

McKinley, M. (Winter 2011). Avoiding a collapse in thinking: Commentary on Jonathan Shedler's "Efficacy of psychodynamic psychotherapy." *Division Review: A Quarterly Psychoanalytic Forum, 1*(1), 28–29.

McWilliams, N. (2004). *Psychoanalytic psychotherapy: A practitioner's guide*. Guilford Press.

Meloy, J. R. (2002). Pathologies of attachment, violence, and criminality. In A. Goldstein (Ed.), *Handbook of psychology: Forensic Psychology* (Vol. 11, pp. 509–26). Wiley.

Meloy, J. R., & Shiva, A. (2007). A psychoanalytic view of the psychopath. In A. Felthous & H. Saß (Eds). *The international handbook of psychopathic disorders and the law* (pp. 335–346). Wiley.

Mikulincer, M., & Shaver, P. R. (2017). Attachment-related contributions to the study of psychopathology. In P. Luyten, L. C. Mayes, P. Fonagy, M. Target, & S. Blatt (Eds.), *Handbook of psychodynamic approaches to psychopathology* (pp. 27–46). Guilford Press.

Morris, D. O., Javier, R. A., & Herron, W. G. (2015). *Specialty competencies in psychoanalysis in psychology*. Oxford University Press.

Muran, J. C. & EuBanks, C. (2020). *Therapist performance under pressure: Negotiating emotions, difference, and rupture*. American Psychological Association.

Munsterberg, H. (1908). *On the witness stand*. Doubleday.

Nesi, D., Garbarino, J., & Prater, C. (2020). Trauma at the heart of forensic developmental psychology. In R. A. Javier, E. A. Owen, & J. A. Maddux (Eds). *Assessing trauma in forensic contexts* (pp. 39–63). Springer.

Nevid, J. S., Rathus, S. A., & Greene, B. (2018/2021). *Abnormal psychology in a changing world*. Pearson.

Nicoli, L., & Bolognini, S. (2022). From *what to how*: A conversation with Stefano Bolognini on emotional attachment. *Psychoanalytic Quarterly, 91*(3), 445–478. doi: 10.1080/00332828.2022.2118502

Offer, D., & Sabshin, M. (Eds.) (1984). *Normality and the life cycle: A critical integration*. Basic Books.

Paniagua, F. A., & Yamada, A. M. (2013). *Handbook of multicultural mental health: Assessment and treatment of diverse populations* (2nd ed.). Elsevier.

Paris, J. (2013). How the history of psychoanalysis interferes with integration. *Journal of Psychotherapy Integration, 23*, 99–106.

Perez-Foster, R. M. (1996). Assessing the psychodynamic function of language in the bilingual patient. In R. M., Perez Foster, M. Moskowitz, & R. A. Javier (Eds.), *Reaching across boundaries of culture and class* (pp. 243–263). Jason Aronson.

Pfabigan, D. M., Seidel, E., Wucherer, A. M., Keckeis, K., Derntl, B., & Lamm, C. (2014). Affective empathy differs in male violent offenders with high- and low-trait psychopathy. *Journal of Personality Disorders, 29*(1), 42–61. https://doi.org/10.1521

Piaget, J. (1995). *The language and thought of the child*. Meridan.

Pine, F. (1990). *Drive, ego, object, and self*. Basic Books.

Pistoia, F., Conson, M., Carolei, A., Dema, M. G., Splendiani, A., Curcio, G., & Sacco, S. (2018). Post-earthquake distress and development of emotional expertise in young adults. *Frontiers in Behavioral Neuroscience, Emotion Regulation and Processing, 12*. https://doi.org/10.3389/fnbeh.2018.00091

Renik, O. (2006). *Practical psychoanalysis for therapists and patients*. Other Press.

Ribot, T. (1891). *The diseases of personality*. Open Court Publishing.

Ribot, T. (1894). *Diseases of the will*. Open Court Publishing.

Ribot, T. (1896). *Diseases of memory: An essay in the positive psychology*. D. Appleton-Century Company.

Rizzuto, A. (2015). *Freud and the spoken word*. Routledge.

Rosen, G. M., & Lilienfield, S. O. (2008). Posttraumatic stress disorder: An empirical evaluation of core assumptions. *Clinical Psychology Review, 28*, 837–868.

Rosenberg, L. M. (2018). Remaining relevant. The application of psychodynamic principles to the mental health workforce. In S. D. Axelrod, P. C. Naso, & L. M. Rosenberg (Eds.), *Papers in psychoanalysis* (pp. 252–272). Routledge.

Rothstein, A. (Ed.) (1985). *Models of the mind: Their relationships to clinical work.* International University Press.

Russell, J. J., Moskowitz, D. S., Zuroff, D. C., Sookman, D., & Paris, J. (2007). Stability and variability of affective experience and interpersonal behavior in borderline personality disorder. *Journal of Abnormal Psychology, 116,* 578–588.

Russell, P. L. (1998a). The role of paradox in repetition compulsion. In J. G. Teicholz & D. Kriegman (Eds.), *Trauma, repetition compulsion, and affect regulation: The work of Paul Russell* (pp. 1–22). Other Press.

Russell, P. L. (1998b). Trauma and the cognitive function of affects. In J. G. Teicholz & D. Kriegman (Eds.). *Trauma, repetition compulsion, and affect regulation: The work of Paul Russell* (pp. 23–47). Other Press.

Safran, J. D. (1998). *Widening the scope of cognitive therapy: The therapeutic relationship, emotion, and the process of change.* Northvale, NJ: Aronson.

Safran, J. (2012). *Psychoanalysis and the psychoanalytic therapies.* American Psychological Association.

Sedler, M. J. (1983). Freud concept of working through. *Psychoanalytic Q., 52*(1), 73–98. PMID:6836082

Shah, G. (2020). Dangerous territory: Racist moments in the psychoanalytic space. *Psychoanalytic Quarterly, 89*(3), 399–418. doi: 10.1080/00332828.2020.1766935

Shedler, J. (2010). The efficacy of psychoanalytic psychotherapy. *American Psychologist, 65*(2), 98–109.

Shedler, J. (2017). Where is the evidence for "evidence-based" therapy? *Journal of Psychological Therapies in Primary Care, 4,* 47–59.

Shulman, M. E. (2021). What use is Freud? *Journal of the American Psychoanalytic Association, 69,* 1093–1113.

Solms, M. & Turnbull, O. (2002). *The brain and the inner world: An introduction to neuroscience of subjective experience.* Other Press.

Solms, M. (2018). Extracts from the revised standard edition of Freud's complete psychological works. *International Journal of Psychoanalysis, 99,* 11–57.

Solms, M. (2021a). A revision of Freud's theory of the biological origins of the Oedipus complex. *The Psychanalytic Quarterly, XC,* 555–581.

Solms, M. (2021b). Revision of drive theory. *Journal of the American Psychoanalytic Association, 69,* 1083–1091.

Solms, M., & Friston, K. (2018). How and why consciousness arises: Some considerations from physics and physiology. *Journal of Consciousness Studies, 25,* 202–208.

Solms, M., & Turnbull, O. (2002). *The brain and the inner world: An introduction to the neuroscience of subjective experience.* Karnac Books.

Solomon, E., & Heide, K. (1999). Type III trauma: Toward a more effective conceptualization of psychological trauma. *International Journal of Offender Therapy and Comparative Criminology, 43,* 202–210.

Steele, M., & Steele, H. (2017). Attachment disorders: In P. Luyten, L. C. Mayes, P. Fonagy, M. Target, & S. Blatt (Eds.), *Handbook of psychodynamic approaches to psychopathology* (pp. 426–444). Guilford Press.

Stern, D. (1985). *The interpersonal world of the infant.* Basic Books.

Stern, D. (1987). Unformulated experience. *Contemporary Psychoanalysis, 19,* 71–99.

Stern, D. B. (2015). *Relational freedom. Emergent properties of the interpersonal field.* Routledge.

Stevens, T., & Morash, M. (2014). Racial/ethnic disparities in boys' probability of arrest and court decisions in 1980 and 2000: The disproportionate impact of "getting tough" on crime. *Youth Violence and Juvenile Justice, 13*(1), 1–19. https://doi.org/10.1177/1541204013515280

Strachey, J. (1893). Charcot: Editor's note. In J. Strachey (Trans.), *The standard edition of the complete psychological works of Sigmund Freud* (Vol. III, pp. 11–23). Hogarth Press.

Sue, D. (2010). *Microaggressions in everyday life.* Wiley.

Sue, D. W., Capodilupo, C. M., Torino, G. C., Bucceri, J. M., Holder, A. M., Nadal, K.L., & Esquilin, M. (2007). Racial microaggression in everyday life: Implications for clinical practice. *American Psychologist, 62*(4), 271–286.

Sullivan, H. S. (1953). *The interpersonal theory of psychiatry.* Norton.

Summers, R. F., & Barber, J. P. (2010). *Psychodynamic therapy. A guide to evidence-based practice.* Guilford Press.

Sutherland, J. D. (1989). Fairbairn's journey into the interior. London: Free Association Books

Thoma, N., Pilecki, B., & McKay, D. (2015). Contemporary cognitive behavior therapy: A review of theory, history, and evidence. *Psychodynamic Psychiatry, 43,* 423–466.

Thompson, C. L. (1996). The African-American patient in psychoanalytic treatment. In R. M. Perez-Foster, M. Moskowitz, & R. A., Javier (Eds.), *Reaching across boundaries of culture and class: Widening the scope of psychotherapy.* Jason Aronson.

Tomkins, S. (1962). *Affect, imagery, consciousness: The positive affects* (Vol. 1). Springer.

Tomkins, S. (1978). Script theory: Differential magnification of affects. In H. E. Howe, Jr., & R. A. Dunstbier (Eds.), *Nebraska symposium on motivation* (pp. 201–236). University of Nebraska Press.

Tuch, R., & Kuttnauer, L. S. (Eds.) (2018). *Conundrums and predicaments in psychotherapy and psychoanalysis.* Routledge.

Tummala-Narra, P. (Ed.) (2021). *Trauma and racial minority immigrants: Turmoil, uncertainty, and resistance.* American Psychological Association.

Vaughans, K. C., & Spielberg, W. (Eds.) (2014). *The psychology of Black boys and adolescents,* (Vol I and II). Praeger.

Verona, E., Sadeh, N., & Javdani, S. (2010). The influences of gender and culture on child and adolescent psychopathy. In R. T. Salekin & D. R. Lynam (Eds.), *Handbook of child and adolescent psychopathy* (pp. 317–342). Guilford Press.

Wachtel, P. L. (1977). *Psychoanalysis and behavior therapy toward an integration.* Basic Books.

Wachtel, P. L. (2010). Beyond "ESTs". Problematic assumptions in the pursuit of evidence-based practice. *Psychoanalytic Psychology, 27,* 251–272.

Wachtel, P. L. (2011). *Therapeutic communication. Knowing what to say when* (2nd ed.). Guilford Press.

Wachtel, P. L. (2014). What must we transcend to make progress in psychoanalysis? Tribal boundaries, the default position, and the self-defeating quest for purity. In S. D. Axelrod, F. C. Naso, & L. M. Rosenberg (Eds.), *Progress in psychoanalysis. Envisioning the future of the profession* (pp. 36–55). Routledge.

Waldinger, R. J., & Schulz, M. S. (2017). Defenses as transdiagnostic window of psychopathology. In P. Luyten, L. C. Mayes, P. Fonagy, M. Target, & S. J. Blatt. (Eds.). *Handbook of psychodynamic approaches to psychopathology* (pp. 110–128). Guilford Press.

Waldron, S., Gazzilo, F., Stukenberg, K., & Gorman, B. S. (2018). Advancing psychoanalysis and psychotherapy through research. In S. D. Axelrod, R. C. Naso, & L. M. Rosenberg

(Eds.), *Progress in psychoanalysis. Envisioning the future of the profession* (pp. 157–180). Routledge.

Wampold, B. E. (2015). How important are the common factors in psychotherapy? An update. *World Psychiatry, 14*, 270–277.

Wampold, B. E., Minami, T. & Baskin, T. W., & Callen Tierney, S. (2002). A Meta (re)analysis of the effects of cognitive therapy versus "other therapies" for depression. *Journal of Affective Disorders, 68*, 159–165.

Wampold, B. E., Mondin, G. W., Moody, M., Stich, F., Benson, K., & Ahn, H. (1997). A meta-analysis of outcome studies comparing bona fide psychotherapies empirically, "all must have prizes." *Psychol. Bull, 122*, 203–215.

Warburton, W., & Anderson, G. A. (2018). On the clinical applications of the general aggression model to understanding domestic violence. In R. A. Javier & W. G. Herron (Eds.), *Understanding domestic violence: Theories, challenges, and remedies* (pp. 71–106). Rowman & Littlefield.

Washington Post Staff. (2018, March 10). Red flags: The troubled path of accused Parkland shooter Nikolas Cruz. https://www.washingtonpost.com/graphics/2018/national/timeline-parkland-shooter-nikolas-cruz/. Retrieved July 28, 2023.

Weinberger, J. & Stoycheva, V. (2020). *The unconscious. Theory, research, and clinical implications*. Guilford Press.

Weiner, I. B., & Bornstein, R. F. (2009). *Principles of psychotherapy: Promoting evidence-based psychodynamic practice*. Wiley.

West, C. M. (2018). Crucial considerations in the understanding and treatment of intimate partner violence in African American couples. In R. A. Javier & W. G. Herron (Eds.). Understanding domestic violence: Theories, challenges, and remedies (pp. 213–235). Rowman & Littlefield.

Western, B., Davis, J., Ganter, & Smith, N. (2021). The cumulative risk of jail incarceration. *Research Article Social Sciences, 118*(16), e2023429118. https://doi.org/10.1073/pnas.2023429118htt8X

Widiger, T. A., & Crego, C. (2018). Mental disorders as discrete clinical conditions: Dimensional versus categorical classification. In D. C. Beidel, & B. C. Frueh (Eds.). *Adult psychopathology and diagnosis* (8th ed., pp. 3–32). Wiley.

Winnicott, D. W. (1965). *The maturational processes and the facilitating environment: Studies in the theory of emotional development*. International University Press.

Winnicott, D. W. (1974). *The maturational processes and the facilitating environment: Studies in the theory of emotional development*. International Universities Press.

Winnicott, D. W. (1986a). *Deprivation and delinquency*. Tavistock.

Winnicott, D. W. (1986b). *Holding and interpretation: Fragment of an analysis*. Grove Press.

Winnicott, D.W. (1988). *Human nature*. Schocken Books.

Wright, J. H., & Davis, D. (1994/2006). The therapeutic relationship in cognitive-behavioral therapy: Patient perceptions and therapists' responses. *Cognitive and Behavioral Practice, 1*(1), 25–45. https://doi.org/10.1016/S1077-7229(05)80085-9

Yakeley, J., & Meloy, J. R. (2012). Understanding violence: Does psychoanalytic thinking matter? *Aggression and Violent Behavior, 17*(3), 229–239.

Yalch, M. (2020). Psychodynamic underpinnings of the DSM-5 alternative model for personality disorder. *Psychoanalytic Psychology, 17*, 219–231.

Yeomans, F. E., Clarkin, J. F., & Kernberg, O. F. (2015). *Transference-focused psychotherapy for borderline personality disorders: A clinical guide*. American Psychiatric Publishing.

Youngstrom, E. C., Prinstein, M. J., Mash, E. J., & Barkley, R. A. (Eds.) (2020). Assessment of disorders in childhood and adolescence. Guilford Press.

Zane, N., Bernal, G., & Leon, F. T. L. (Ed.) (2016). *Evidence-based psychological practice with ethnic minorities: Culturally-informed research and clinical strategies.* American Psychological Association. http://dx.doi.org/10.1037/14940-001

Zayas, L. (2015). *Forgotten citizens: Deportation, children and the making of American exiles and orphans.* Oxford University Press.

Zilcha-Mano, S. (2017). Is the alliance really therapeutic? Revisiting this question in light of recent methodological advances. *American Psychologist, 72,* 311–325.

Zuckerman, M. (2003). Are there racial and ethnic differences in psychopathic personality? A critique of Lynn's (2002) racial and ethnic differences in psychopathic personality. *Personality and Individual Differences, 5*(6), 1463–1469.

Index

About the Authors

William G. Herron is a supervisor in the Psychiatric Residency Program at Bergen New Bridge Medical Center and in independent practice in Woodcliff Lake, New Jersey. He was professor in the Clinical Psychology Program at St. John's University for forty years and director of Clinical Psychology and of School Psychology during his time there. He was also Faculty, Supervisor, Training Analyst, and Clinical Director at the Contemporary Center for Advanced Psychoanalytic Studies and at the New Jersey Institute for Psychoanalytic Training where he was Training Board Chair. He has authored, coauthored, or coedited fourteen books, primarily with a psychodynamic emphasis, as well as numerous articles. His frequent collaborator is Rafael Javier. His most recent book was *Understanding Domestic Violence* (2018), and his most recent article was "The Impact of Pluralism" (2019) published in *Psychology and Psychological Research International Journal*.

Rafael Art. Javier is a professor of Psychology and the director of the Post-Graduate Professional Development Programs and the Postdoctoral Certificate Programs in Forensic Psychology at St. John's University. He is a faculty and supervisor at the Object Relations Institute and the New York University Postdoctoral Program in Psychotherapy and Psychoanalysis. He is a founding member of the Center of Latin American and Caribbean Studies (CLAS) and the first founding Director of the Center for Psychological Services and Clinical Studies at St. John's University for almost twenty years. Dr. Javier has presented at national and international conferences on psycholinguistic and psychoanalytic issues in research and treatment and on ethnic and cultural issues in psychoanalytic theories and practice, including on issues of violence and the impact on general cognitive and emotional functioning. He has published extensively on the subject including several coedited books. His current research includes issues of violence and the nature of autobiographical memory and bilingualism, particularly related to traumatic memories. His most recent books include *Understanding Domestic Violence: Theories, Challenges, Remedies*, coedited with William Herron, and *Assessing Trauma in Forensic Contexts*, coedited with Drs. Elizabeth Owen and Jemour Maddux. He is the editor-in-chief of the *Journal of Psycholinguistic Research* and on the editorial board of the *Journal of Psycholinguistic Research*, the *Journal of Social Distress and the Homeless*, and the *Journal of Infant, Child, and Adolescent Psychotherapy*. He was the 2017–2018 President of the Forensic Division of the New York State Psychological Association and the past vice president of the Association of Hispanic Mental Health Professionals. He is a Fellow of the American Psychological Association.